T0144682

BASIC HEALTH PUBLICATIONS USER'S GUIDE

TO THE Top 10 Natural Therapies

Your Introductory Guide to the Best That Natural and Alternative Therapies Offer

Marcus Laux, N.D.
& Melissa Block, M.Ed.

JACK CHALLEM Series Editor

The information contained in this book is based upon the research and personal and professional experiences of the authors. It is not intended as a substitute for consulting with your physician or other healthcare provider. Any attempt to diagnose and treat an illness should be done under the direction of a healthcare professional.

The publisher does not advocate the use of any particular healthcare protocol but believes the information in this book should be available to the public. The publisher and authors are not responsible for any adverse effects or consequences resulting from the use of the suggestions, preparations, or procedures discussed in this book. Should the reader have any questions concerning the appropriateness of any procedures or preparations mentioned, the authors and the publisher strongly suggest consulting a professional healthcare advisor.

Series Editor: Jack Challem
Editor: Roberta W. Waddell
Typesetter: Gary A. Rosenberg
Series Cover Designer: Mike Stromberg

Basic Health Publications User's Guides are published by Basic Health Publications, Inc.

CONTENTS

Introduction

Nearly two and a half centuries ago, the Greek physician Hippocrates coined the phrase *vis medicatrix naturae:* the healing power of nature. This principle describes the body's intrinsic tendency to heal. This connection that doctoring once had with the natural world is all but lost now. Conventional physicians are trained in the use of pharmacological agents and high-tech diagnostic and surgical procedures, but not in the practice of natural healing.

On the other hand, consumers are interested in natural therapies these days and they are pushing mainstream medicine in that direction. In fact, about 50 percent of Americans incorporate some form of complementary or alternative medicine (CAM) into their health care. They're not only looking to get rid of an illness today, they're looking for a healing path that will boost their overall health for life.

Traditional (Natural) Medicine in the Information Age

It's not easy to find reliable information on the various natural therapies that are currently available. Public interest in natural alternatives has outpaced modern clinical research into those alternatives. Although the medical establishment is doing its best to keep up—two-thirds of American medical schools now offer courses in CAM, and the federal government has created the National Center for Complementary and Alternative Medicine (NCCAM)—there is still a need for unbiased, high-quality information on natural therapies.

The government does not regulate nutritional supplements the way it does drugs, and along with all the genuine suppliers, the door is open to hucksters willing to bend the truth to sell a product. Contradictory information abounds. The two of us—a naturopathic physician with extensive knowledge of natural medicine and extensive modalities and a health journalist who has authored and coauthored dozens of books on these topics—have written this guide to help you make sense of the best approaches and to give you guidance about how to pursue the ones that most appeal to you.

Promise and Problems of Contemporary Medicine

The lightning-quick movement that Western medical science made into its current state has brought both promise and problems. At times, mainstream medicine does more harm than good. It is estimated that some 180,000 people die each year due to *iatrogenic injury*—injury caused by medical treatment. An estimated 106,000 of those deaths are due to the adverse effects of drugs, not to any error on the part of doctors or hospitals (except in originally prescribing them). Unnecessary surgery is believed to be the cause of some 12,000 deaths a year, and medical errors are thought to cause 7,000 deaths per year. Countless thousands of others experience adverse drug effects and iatrogenic injuries that don't kill, but do reduce the quality of life.

Illnesses that today's medicine cannot cure, treat effectively, or even fully understand—including allergies, asthma, autoimmune diseases, cancer, chronic fatigue syndrome, diabetes, environmental illness, fibromyalgia, irritable bowel syndrome, and some psychological disorders—are on the rise. People who have these diseases are often told by establishment medicine

Chronic Disease
Any disease state that can be controlled but not cured, that is not expected to improve, and that lasts a lifetime or recurs.

that their only option is symptom-control with drugs. Most are not told it's possible to find a healing path through natural medicine.

The current system of sick care places too heavy a reliance on doctors and health insurers instead of asking each person to take better care of him- or herself. Self-care is a big part of natural medicine, and in order for natural medicine to work its best, people have to actively participate and make knowledgeable choices. This book will help you do just that.

What Is a Natural Therapy, and Why Is It Better?

The term *natural* can be misleading. When you take a tablet made up of ascorbic acid—vitamin C—the vitamin in that tablet is identical to the vitamin C you find in oranges and hot peppers. Those vitamin-C molecules are all identical in structure, and your body can't tell the difference between them. But the vitamin-C supplement is made from molecules that have been synthesized in a laboratory, while the vitamin C found in oranges and hot peppers comes straight from Mother Nature's pharmacy.

When we use the word *natural* in regard to nutrients, hormones, and other substances discussed in this book, what we mean is that it is *identical* to something that is found in nature. Many of the natural therapies we discuss in this book don't come straight from the natural world. We can still call them natural, however, because when placed under a microscope, they are indistinguishable from the real thing.

Allopathic medicines are often derived from natural substances, but are then tweaked to increase their potency and specificity. Changing their molecular

Allopathy
Technologically advanced, specialized Western medicine, currently the dominant method of treatment; treats the symptoms of disease rather than getting to the root of the problem in the whole person.

structure this way allows the drugmakers to patent and sell them at whatever exorbitant price they wish for at least seventeen years. Drugmakers are, therefore, much more motivated to research, create, and sell synthetic drugs than they are to market substances from nature, which are generally not patentable.

The specificity of single, highly isolated synthetic drugs can affect the body in ways that cause significant adverse effects. It's not possible to target and change one small aspect of the body, which is made up of several interdependent systems, without these kinds of repercussions. Natural therapies, on the other hand, have a broader, gentler, less intense action that works with the body's intricate symphony, and they are associated with fewer and milder side effects.

Another problem with highly targeted drug therapy is that, with many disease processes, there isn't yet a good enough understanding of their causes to figure out exactly what should be targeted. Such conditions as allergies, asthma, autoimmune disease, cancer, diabetes, and heart disease, are *multifactorial*—they have many contributory factors, not all of which medical science currently understands and cannot therefore address broadly enough, whereas natural medicine works at many levels to address many of these factors.

And, finally, drug therapy is usually only a temporary fix. People with chronic diseases are led to believe that, despite the unpleasant side effects, they will have to be on prescription medications for life in order to control their condition. Once the drugs are stopped, the illness returns, unlike natural therapies, which are aimed at actually reversing the course of these illnesses and restoring health.

The Best of Both Worlds

Mainstream and natural medical approaches work best when they are used as part of a continuum, with natural healing methods used to support opti-

mal health and aid recovery from chronic or mild illnesses, and allopathy reserved for times when more
dramatic interventions for life-threatening crises are
necessary. When used in this kind of complementary way, the strengths of each approach can help to
compensate for the weaknesses of the other.

When your health problems are chronic and not
life-threatening, you can rely almost exclusively on
natural approaches. More serious illnesses may require allopathic treatments, but you can usually complement those treatments with supportive natural
ones. And once you're healthy again, you can lean
more on natural medicine to keep you that way.

A natural therapy can be:

- Whole plants or foods (herbs, medicinal mushrooms, and superfoods), which are used more or
  less as they are found in nature;

- Derived from plants or other substances in nature,
  maintaining the overall molecular structure and
  chemistry of those plants; or it can be *standardized*—ensuring that the plant extract contains
  predictable amounts of health-promoting phytochemicals (plant chemicals);

- A remedy that employs natural substances, or
  hands-on therapy, such as bodywork, massage,
  or adjustments, to help people heal or stay well;

- A substance that is synthesized in a lab and pro-
  duced in a factory, but is molecularly identical to
  a substance found in nature.

Whether you are currently
well and want to stay that way,
or are trying to heal from an
illness, you will find answers in
the pages of this book, which
contains chapters on healing
diets and superfoods, nutritional supplements, herbal
medicine, homeopathy, chiro-

Naturopathy
*A medical approach
to good health that
utilizes natural medicines
and natural therapies,
and treats the whole
person.*

practic and osteopathic manipulation, massage and other kinds of bodywork, spirituality and mind/body work, Ayurvedic medicine, acupuncture and traditional Chinese medicine, and naturopathy. In this highly focused guide, you'll learn enough about all these topics to truly take charge of your own health.

CHAPTER 1

HEALING DIETS AND SUPERFOODS

The basic foundation of any healthy lifestyle is a good diet made up primarily of nutrient-dense vegetables, fruits, whole grains, beans, beneficial fats, and lean protein, and goes easy on saturated fat and sugar. There are many variations on the theme of healthy eating—specific diets that come and go with much hullabaloo and are promoted as the newest and best dietary revolution—until the next fad comes along, that is. Beyond these over-hyped diets are those designed to heal the body in a more aggressive way—to reverse disease or slow the aging process.

We will avoid the fad diets altogether, and focus instead on those diets and individual foods—the *superfoods*—that are forms of natural medicine. These dietary approaches to healing are tried and true over the course of history, a testament to Hippocrates' oft-quoted wisdom: "Let your food be your medicine, and your medicine your food."

If your health is generally good, and your diet is nutritious and well-balanced, and includes a few superfoods on a regular basis, there's no need for you to follow the more extreme diets in this chapter. If you have eaten a poor diet for years—and you know who you are—and/or are suffering from chronic disease, such as allergies, arthritis, asthma, an autoimmune disease, cancer, diabetes, or heart disease, a more extreme approach may suit you better.

If you are extremely ill or are undergoing aggressive medical treatment for any of the above conditions, you may well benefit from one of the more stringent diet plans in this chapter, but you *must not use those plans without the guidance of your healthcare practitioner.*

Your Basic Healing Diet— Whole Organic Foods

The easiest way to get your general health moving in a better direction is to adopt a whole foods diet. Eat things that come from nature, not from a bag, box, can, or microwaveable container.

The basis of the whole-foods diet is a combination of vegetables, fruit, and whole grains. (Whole grains are minimally processed so they maintain their nutritious, fiber-rich husks.) Add to this small amounts of healthy oils—extra-virgin olive, organic butter, avocado or coconut oils—and moderate servings of lean protein, particularly deepwater, coldwater fish, such as mackerel, salmon, halibut, and sardines. Free-range organic eggs, free-range organic poultry, grass-fed beef, and tofu and tempeh are other good protein sources for the whole-foods diet. Cook vegetables, meats, and fish by baking, steaming, roasting, poaching, blanching, stir-frying, or sautéing; avoid deep-frying, and grill only occasionally (it causes the production of carcinogens in meats). Microwaving is all right in a pinch.

Eat some raw vegetables and fruit every day for the enzymes they contain in the raw state. And, if you enjoy them, cooked and/or sprouted beans— adzuki, black, garbanzo, kidney, navy, pinto, or white—are all healthy eating.

If you like dairy products, use organic versions without added sugar, and use them in moderation. If you can't live without bread, bagels, and pasta, try wholegrain or sprouted-grain versions. You'll come to appreciate their heartier taste and texture.

Drink at least eight 8-ounce glasses of pure, clean water each day. Herbal teas are good too. If you like juices, go the fresh-squeezed route. Red wine is rich in powerful antioxidant substances that have been linked with longer life and that help prevent heart disease and cancer, but drink no more than one to two glasses of wine, or one beer, per day. Limit your coffee consumption to one or two cups a day and stick with the organic variety. Non-organic coffee is treated with fungicides, pesticides, and other unsavory chemicals, then roasted—not good!

How about desserts and *no-no* snack foods? Use them infrequently, and go for quality, not quantity. Have one scoop of quality ice cream instead of a hot fudge sundae. Buy a small bar of organic dark chocolate that's loaded with healthful antioxidants and eat it slowly instead of wolfing down a king-sized Snickers bar. Bake cookies from scratch, eat one or two yourself, and give the rest away.

If you shift from fast food, processed foods, and sugar to this kind of whole-foods diet, you'll move into better health. You'll be eating fewer calories, more fiber, and more vitamins and minerals. Your digestive function will improve and your energy level will soar. If you're battling chronic disease, you may find less need for drugs as your symptoms are reduced.

Cleansing Diets

Why cleansing diets? Because life is now lived in a soup of synthetic chemicals—they appear in the foods we eat, the air we breathe, and the insides of homes and workplaces. Many toxic chemicals have been found stored away in the tissues of people and animals across the globe. Because of the ways in which these substances spread and bioaccumulate (collect in larger and larger concentrations as they move up the food chain), it appears there isn't a creature or an ecosystem anywhere on the planet that is unaffected. Research has shown that many of these chemicals are carcinogenic (cancer-causing or cancer-promoting) or harmful to reproductive health.

Many experts have theorized that toxic chemicals are a cause—if not *the* cause—of many chronic health problems. Consider, too, that foreign chemicals are introduced into the body when prescription and over-the-counter drugs are ingested. Further, the body *naturally* produces toxins in the course of immune-system activity and metabolism.

The body can get rid of these toxins through several avenues, notably the intestines, the skin, the urinary tract, and the liver, lungs, throat, lymph, and sinus systems. Cleansing diets support all these natural eliminative functions.

Examples of Cleansing Diets

Any of the cleansing diets and fasts described in this chapter can be followed for a minimum of three days, and all of them are safe for as long as a month (as long as you are generally healthy and not pregnant or breastfeeding). Ideally, you will adopt one of these diets two to four times a year or more, to help jump-start natural cleansing and to break away from any addictions to refined foods and sugar.

The most basic, and the easiest, of these diets consists of fresh vegetables and fruit, both raw and cooked, along with whole grains, either cooked or sprouted. Water, freshly pressed juices, and herbal teas are allowed. This is about as extreme as you should get if you are pregnant or breastfeeding. If you are actively being treated for a chronic illness, check with your nutritionally educated healthcare practitioner before moving on to the next level of cleansing.

This next level is vegetables and fruits only. At this level and further along, you may experience what's known as a *healing crisis*—because your body is rebalancing, healing energy is stimulated, and waste and toxins are being removed. This may lead you to experience a headache, fatigue, nausea, rash, or other symptoms. You can minimize this by eating a healthy, low-sugar, high-nutrient diet in the days before your cleansing diet. Before the diet or fast, spend half as many days eating a wholesome, whole-foods diet, and gradually work back into that diet after your cleanse, before going back to your usual fare (if you even want to after tasting how delicious whole unprocessed foods can be).

> A few thousand milligrams of vitamin C per day can help you weather a healing crisis.

Next in the cleansing-diet spectrum come raw foods. A raw-food diet consists of nothing but raw foods, water, and freshly pressed juices. Raw foods are living food—their enzymes and other synergistic ingredients promote digestion and revitalize the body. And raw-food diets can be delicious. Resources abound for aspiring raw-foodists who want to keep their diets interesting. And learning to "cook" raw will help you incorporate more raw food into your daily fare, long-term.

You can eat sprouted beans and grains, soaked or sprouted raw nuts, and as many fresh uncooked vegetables and fruits as you like. Try cheeses and yogurts made from seeds instead of dairy.

> Do not put any child or teen on a low-calorie diet without first consulting a nutritionally aware healthcare practitioner for guidance.

Macrobiotics

Macrobiotics—from the Greek *makro*, for long, and *bios*, for life—is more than a diet. It's a lifestyle, the art and science of health and longevity.

The macrobiotic diet consists of whole grains, such as brown rice, millet, oats, and spelt (40 to 60 percent); leafy greens and other vegetables (20 to 30 percent); and sea vegetables (seaweed) and beans (combined, about 5 to 10 percent). One to two servings of white fish or other seafood per week may be included. Roasted or raw nuts and seeds may be eaten as snacks.

Macrobiotics encourages relaxed, orderly eating, and gratitude for what you consume. It is recommended that you chew your food very thoroughly—50 times per mouthful—and that you eat until you are about 80-percent full. Eating within three hours of bedtime is not recommended.

Many have attributed their healing from diseases they had previously been unable to cure—including cancer, diabetes, and heart disease—to the macrobiotic diet. You can find success stories on the website of the Kushi Institute, the premier center for macrobiotic education in the United States: www.kushiinstitute.org.

Superfoods

If advertisers are going to employ the influence of superheroes to sell foods to the public, they should represent the superfoods too—foods that, in their natural form, offer wide-ranging and scientifically proven health benefits. Studies of populations throughout the world have shown that eating these foods often translates to better health, longer life, and increased resistance to disease.

Allium Vegetables

This class of vegetables includes garlic, leeks, onions, and shallots—foods unrivalled as flavorings. Allium vegetables have been folk remedies for colds, flus, and infections since the earliest days of natural medicine. They are rich in sulfur compounds that have potent detoxifying and anti-cancer effects.

Berries

Scientists believe one of the main disease-fighting ingredient in blueberries and other deeply colored berries, such as cranberries, strawberries, and goji, a type of berry found at high altitudes in Asia (you can find dried goji berries and goji juice on the Internet), is a class of plant chemicals known as *anthocyanidins*. These chemicals decrease the risk of cardiovascular disease, improve vision, and help prevent cancer by quenching free radicals and inducing cancer-cell death (apoptosis). Blueberries and cranberries are also helpful natural treatments for urinary tract infection.

Recent research at Tufts University found that a blueberry-rich diet helped aging rats navigate mazes faster and maintain a more youthful balance and coordination. Animals genetically engineered to develop Alzheimer's-like plaques in their brains showed less of this damage when fed blueberries. Blueberry phytochemicals help nerve cells (neurons) in aging brains communicate better with one another. Tufts researcher James Joseph, M.D., has been so convinced by his own research that he eats one to two cups of blueberries a day. You can eat the berries fresh or dried, but your best bet is wild blueberries, which have more antioxidant power than cultivated blueberries.

Cruciferous Vegetables

Of all the cruciferous vegetables—broccoli, Brussels sprouts, cabbage, cauliflower, and kale—broccoli is the richest natural source of three important chemicals, indole-3-carbinol (I-3-C), diindolylmethane (DIM), and sulforaphane, all of which can stop cancer cold in laboratory and animal studies. Current research suggests that broccoli protects against stomach cancer by helping to kill off antibiotic-resistant *H. pylori*, the bug implicated in most cases of stomach ulcers, whose presence has been linked with stomach cancer. All the crucifers are rich in compounds that enhance the liver's detoxification of carcinogens, and overall research shows that people who eat lots of crucifers are protecting themselves against breast and prostate cancer, among others.

Flaxseeds

These tiny brown seeds are a rich source of alpha-linolenic acid, an anti-inflammatory, brain-boosting omega-3 fat. Flax is also rich in lignans, a type of soluble (digestible) fiber that can bring down cholesterol and post-meal blood sugar. Supplementing with flaxseeds can decrease blood markers of inflammation, improve gastrointestinal health, and possibly reduce the risk for colon cancer.

Buy whole flaxseeds and grind them as needed with a coffee grinder. If you use flax oil, your best bet is organic, high-lignan oil, in a black bottle to prevent light-induced oxidation.

Green Foods

Chlorella and spirulina algae are extremely efficient at transmuting the sun's energy into nutrients. Of all the plants, these are the richest natural source of chlorophyll, the plant chemical that performs this alchemical transformation of energy into nutrients, and is an excellent internal cleanser and detoxifier. Green foods are rich in omega-3 fats and vitamin B_{12}, and are a good way for those not fond of vegetables to add to their daily ration of green.

Try broken-cell-wall chlorella, spirulina, or barley or wheat grass, or any combination. They are used as supplements or juiced.

Leafy Greens

Spinach and other leafy greens—beet greens, chard, collard greens, kohlrabi, mustard greens, and turnip greens—protect against cataracts and age-related macular degeneration, as well as cancers of the colon, esophagus, lung, oral cavity, pancreas, stomach, throat, and uterus. Spinach is the richest food source of lutein and zeaxanthin, carotenoid nutrients that help block ultraviolet radiation and keep it from damaging the eyes and are highly recommended for eye health. Eat leafy greens often, raw or cooked.

Medicinal Mushrooms

Maitake, reishi, and shiitake mushrooms have been integral parts of traditional Chinese and Japanese medicine for centuries. They are rich in compounds that heighten immunity against cancer and infectious diseases. Research shows they are useful for cancer prevention and, for those already fighting the disease, they help minimize the harsh effects of chemotherapy.

Both fresh and dried shiitake mushrooms are widely available and they make a delicious addition to soups, stews, and stir-fries. You can shop for medicinal mushrooms in your local market, or purchase them dried through mail order (*see* the resources section).

Salmon (Wild)

This fish has delicate flavor, ruby-pink flesh, and rich stores of the heart-and brain-protective omega-3 fats EPA (eicosapentaenoic acid) and DHA (docosahexaenoic acid). At its worst, when salmon is grown in a fish farm, its flesh is greyish-pink, tasteless, and full of dieldrin, dioxins, PCBs, and toxaphene—all potentially harmful to human health.

There is an enormous difference between wild and farmed salmon. If you've never tried wild salmon (usually labeled as such), you can't say you have ever really experienced this food. Farmed salmon is fed an unnatural diet that does not contain the natural pink pigment (astaxanthin) abundant in salmon's natural ocean diet. Farmed salmon are given antibiotics to prevent infections caused by overcrowding and poor diet. Avoid farmed fish (this includes Atlantic salmon). Wild salmon's color is different, but be careful because a recent study found that many merchants are trying to pass farmed salmon off as wild. To be sure, you can buy wild salmon, or other fish, such as sablefish, sardines, and tuna, online at www.vitalchoice.com.

Tea

Green tea contains flavonoids that help blood-vessel walls remain flexible and reduce the stickiness of blood platelets. Test-tube studies show that tea flavonoids—black and green—inhibit tumor formation. Tea drinkers have a lower risk of cancers of the esophagus, liver, lung, mouth, pancreas, prostate, skin, small intestine, and stomach. Tea may even prevent tooth decay. Try decaffeinated herbal teas, and try green tea (which has some caffeine) or breakfast teas to perk you up in the morning. Peppermint or ginger tea can soothe gastrointestinal distress, while chamomile tea can help you relax.

Tomatoes

Lycopene, a carotenoid nutrient found abundantly in tomatoes, inhibits prostate cancer. It reduces DNA damage (the first step in carcinogenesis) in the prostate, and increases the body's production of anti-inflammatory and antioxidant substances. In test-tube and animal studies, it helps the liver neutralize carcinogens.

Lycopene may help prevent breast cancer. Higher intake of lycopene from papayas, pink grapefruits, pink guavas, tomatoes, and watermelons is associated with a lowered risk of heart disease and strokes. To improve lycopene absorption, eat tomatoes cooked with oil.

Yogurt

Milk with added friendly bacteria—*lactobacillus acidophilus, lactobacillus bulgaricus,* and *streptococcus thermophilus*—curdles as its sugars are transformed into lactic acid, a culturing that was probably invented as a form of preservation. Yogurt has long been a staple of diets in Asia, Southeastern Europe, and the Middle East, and worldwide studies show that people who regularly consume yogurt have longer lives and fewer chronic diseases.

Yogurt helps correct constipation, diarrheal diseases, *H. pylori* infection, inflammatory bowel disease, and lactose intolerance by re-establishing the proper balance of bacterial good guys and bad guys in the gut—a balance often knocked askew by antibiotic drugs, birth control pills, stress, or diets rich in refined flours and sugars. This intestinal balance is believed to play an important role in the prevention of colon cancer and yeast overgrowth (candidiasis). Eat unsweetened live-culture yogurt, adding a little fruit, honey, jam, or maple syrup for flavor, if desired. Or use plain yogurt in place of sour cream.

By including these superfoods in your diet as often as possible, you'll be increasing your odds of living a long healthy life free of disease and disability. Other foods—avocadoes, citrus fruits, oats, pumpkin seeds, and walnuts, for example—could definitely be understudies to the culinary heroes on this list, but we have addressed some the major players in the superfood drama that can promote better health.

Healing Diet Reality Check

The bottom line: Eat food as close to its natural form as possible; avoid processed foods, sugar, and toxic chemical additives; stick with fat sources, such as olive oil, that have established health benefits; and maintain balance and variety in your daily fare. Beyond that, fine-tune to suit your tastes, your lifestyle, and any condition you are trying to heal.

For resources and more information, turn to the resources section.

CHAPTER 2

NUTRITIONAL SUPPLEMENTS

Most Americans regularly use at least one nutritional supplement—the daily multivitamin. It's a form of health insurance, watching your back when there isn't time or energy to eat nutritious food. There is convincing evidence that even the healthiest foods are less nourishing than they once were because soils are depleted and foods are raised and grown in unnatural ways. In a world filled with toxic chemicals and equally toxic stress, it makes sense to boost your defenses against disease with a daily multivitamin/mineral combination.

Some supplements go beyond the basic day-to-day requirements and target biochemical processes that need balancing, boosting, or other kinds of support. Integrative physicians and other natural healthcare practitioners can skillfully use individual nutrients to help people who are ill move back toward balanced health. In this chapter, you'll learn how to create your own basic supplement program.

Over- or Undernutrition

Macronutrients
Nutrient substances, including carbohydrates, fats, protein, fiber, and water, that are needed in large amounts in order to maintain optimum health.

In developing nations, millions of people don't get enough to eat, resulting in severe nutrient deficiencies and taking a toll beyond the comprehension of the average person. On the other side of the spectrum are Westerners who are definitely *not* lacking, at least not in macronutrients. With the prevalence of overweight and obesity at about 65 percent in the United States, Americans are getting plenty of calories from too much refined sugar and fat.

Unfortunately, many people do not have an adequate daily intake of the essential vitamins and minerals, which are found most abundantly in deeply colored vegetables, legumes, and fruits, and whole grains. Nutrition experts have long pressed Americans to get their five servings of these essential food groups every day, but only 20 or 30 percent are meeting these goals.

Over the years, a lack of nutrients can evolve into *subclinical* deficiency that can predispose people to chronic and age-related diseases. A great deal of research has confirmed this link between poor micronutrient nutrition and the risk of cancer, heart disease, and death from all causes:

Micronutrients
Vitamins or minerals that the body must obtain from outside sources; these nutrients are essential to the body in small amounts.

- People whose diets lack folate and vitamins B_6 and B_{12} are at greater risk for heart attacks, strokes, and possibly Alzheimer's disease. These nutrients are required for the breakdown of *homocysteine*, an amino acid (a component of protein) that is toxic to the walls of blood vessels when it accumulates.

- A low intake of antioxidant nutrients—including vitamins C and E, and the accessory nutrients (which are described in more detail below) beta-carotene, flavonoids, lycopene, and others—has been linked to an increased risk for cancer and heart disease.

Accessory Nutrients
Health-promoting nutrients, not vitamins or minerals, not required for life. Although the body makes some, they are most beneficial in the greater amounts found in foods or supplements.

- It has been estimated that about 32 percent of the cancer deaths in the United States could be prevented through dietary modification by increasing the intake of fruits, vegetables, and whole grains—all rich sources of vitamins, minerals, and accessory nutrients.

The Basics of Daily Vitamin and Mineral Supplements

Vitamins
Substances that help drive the machinery of cellular function; many affect immune function and act as antioxidants, guarding the body against toxic free radicals.

Vitamin labels now list a daily value (DV), the current evolution of the former recommended daily allowance (RDA). Nutrients that aren't essential, or required in the diet, are listed as an adequate intake (AI) or come with a note that the nutrient is non-essential. The following sections set forth the DVs for each nutrient. Some multis will contain a bit more or less than the values listed here. If you decide to take a higher dosage than that found in the multi, add additional supplements on to it. (These values are for adults.)

Minerals
Elements originating in the earth; cannot be made by living systems; work as coenzymes in biochemical reactions; build bone, contract and release muscles, generate nerve impulses, and support immune function.

If we make no recommendation separate from the DV, we are recommending the DV as a safe dosage. When we specify conditions for which the nutrient may be therapeutic, we are usually referring to dosages on the higher end of the spectrum. To use vitamins or minerals as specific disease treatments, confer with a healthcare professional who is nutritionally savvy.

Vitamin A

- Immune boosting, needed for eye health; may be toxic at high doses (above 10,000 IU) if taken for months.
- Daily value (DV): 5,000 IU

  May be good for: Improving night vision, skin health, immune-system function

Vitamin B$_1$ (Thiamin)

- This and other B vitamins are important for cellular metabolism, nervous system function, and skin health
- DV: 1.5 mg
- Therapeutic dose: 50–200 mg

May be good for: Confusion, dementia, depression, fatigue, neuropathy, pain

Vitamin B$_2$ (Riboflavin)

- DV: 1.7 mg
- Therapeutic dose: 50–200 mg

May be good for: Chronic alcohol or drug use, fatigue, thyroid and adrenal gland health, dry skin, depression

Vitamin B$_3$ (Niacin)

- DV: 20 mg
- Therapeutic dose: 50–200 mg

May be good for: Depression, diabetes, intermittent claudication, memory impairment, osteoarthritis, rheumatoid arthritis

Vitamin B$_5$ (Pantothenic Acid)

- DV: 10 mg
- Therapeutic dose: 50–250 mg

May be good for: Adrenal gland dysfunction, allergies, fatigue, high triglyceride levels, infections, rheumatoid arthritis, ulcerative colitis

Vitamin B$_6$ (Pyridoxine)

- DV: 2 mg
- Therapeutic dose: 30–250 mg

May be good for: Asthma, autism, carpal tunnel syndrome, depression, diabetes, eczema, heart disease, kidney stones, osteoporosis, PMS, pregnancy-related nausea

Vitamin B$_{12}$

- DV: 6 mcg
- Therapeutic dose: 1,000–5,000 mcg

May be good for: AIDS, anemia, asthma, dementia, depression, epilepsy, fatigue, hepatitis, infertility, multiple sclerosis, neuropathy, numbness, psychosis, tingling, tinnitus; injected, intranasal, or sublingual may work better

Biotin

- A vitamin in the B group
- DV: 300 mcg
- Therapeutic dose: 1,000–5,000 mcg

May be good for: Brittle nails, dandruff, fatigue, hair loss (caused by biotin deficiency), muscle weakness, scaly yellow skin lesions, type 2 diabetes

Folic Acid

- Also a B vitamin
- DV: 400 mcg
- Therapeutic dose: 400–1,000 mcg

May be good for: Cancer prevention, high homocysteine (risk factor for Alzheimer's, heart disease), macrocytic anemia (sign of folate deficiency), mood disorders, prevention of neural tube defects

Vitamin C

- Immune boosting, component of connective tissue
- DV: 600 mg
- Therapeutic dose: 200–2,000 mg

May be good for: Chronic infection, fatigue, gingivitis, low immunity, poor wound healing

Vitamin D

- Bone health, possible anti-cancer nutrient; made in body during ultraviolet light exposure; taking too much orally can damage liver
- DV: 400 IU

May be good for: Bone strength in people of all ages who don't get enough sun

Vitamin E

- Antioxidant, helps prevent excess blood clotting, may lower risk of cancer and heart disease
- DV: 30 IU
- Therapeutic dose: 200–400 IU

May be good for: Fatigue, high stress, risk of heart disease, susceptibility to infection

Vitamin K

- Affects blood clotting and may reduce heart attack risk; made by intestinal bacteria, bone formation
- DV: 80 mcg
- Therapeutic dose: 100–500 mcg

May be good for: Heavy periods, osteoporosis prevention

Calcium

- This mineral builds and strengthens bone, and is integral in muscle-cell activity and blood-pressure regulation
- DV: 1,000 mg
- Therapeutic dose: 800–1,200 mg

May be good for: Bone health, hypertension, muscle spasms and twitches

Chromium

- This mineral has been studied in depth for its blood-sugar-lowering effects
- DV: 120 mcg
- Therapeutic dose: 50–200 mcg

May be good for: Carbohydrate addiction, pre-diabetes, type 2 diabetes

Copper

- Important building block of connective tissue; also needed for oxygen transport in the bloodstream and production of superoxide dismutase, an antioxidant enzyme
- DV: 2 mg

May be good for: Osteoporosis, rheumatoid arthritis

Iron

- This mineral should be taken primarily by premenopausal women
- DV: 18 mg

May be good for: Anemia

Iodine

- A trace mineral needed for thyroid health
- DV: 150 mg

May be good for: Goiter, pregnancy-related thyroid dysfunction, thyroid function

Manganese

- This mineral is important for blood clotting, metabolism of cholesterol and protein, normal bone growth, and producing enzymes for building connective tissues
- DV: 2 mg

May be good for: Diabetes, epileptic seizures, osteoporosis

Magnesium

- Important for bone, circulatory, and respiratory health
- DV: 400 mg
- Therapeutic dose: 600 mg

May be good for: Asthma, heart disease, osteoporosis, spasms

Molybdenum

- This trace mineral plays a role in liver detoxification and in maintaining a healthy urinary tract
- DV: 75 mcg

May be good for: Esophageal cancer, improved dental health (fewer cavities are found in people with higher intake of this mineral)

Phosphorus

- Needed for healthy bones; doses higher than the DV can cause calcium loss
- DV: 1,000 mg

May be good for: Osteoporosis prevention, increasing energy

Potassium

- This mineral helps regulate blood pressure and body fluid levels, and helps to free up stored carbohydrates when needed for energy
- DV: 4,000 mg

May be good for: helping to compensate for potassium loss with heart-failure drugs, kidney stone prevention, and prevention of irregular heartbeat (arrhythmia) and hypertension

Selenium

- Believed to protect against several cancers and heart disease, and to enhance immunity; powerful antioxidant
- DV: 70 mcg
- Therapeutic dose: 70–200 mcg

May be good for: Cancer prevention, fatigue, inflammatory disorders, recurrent infections

Zinc

- Boosts immunity, aids in wound healing, strengthens bones, improves skin and prostate health
- DV: 15 mg

- Therapeutic dose: Up to 150 mg (higher doses can hamper immune function)

May be good for: Colds, flu, prostate enlargement, fertility, dry skin, poor immune function

Accessory Nutrients to Consider Supplementing

Accessory nutrients, such as alpha lipoic acid, bioflavonoids, carotenoids, coenzyme Q_{10}, fiber, and omega-3 fatty acids have important, diverse functions. Some aid in better gastrointestinal function, some are cogs in the machinery of cellular energy production, some help decrease inflammation, while others support immune function, and still others work as antioxidants, protecting the body against free-radical damage.

These nutrients can be used to round out a basic supplement plan, or they can be used medicinally in higher doses. If you plan to do the latter, your best bet is to consult with a trained and knowledgable doctor or healthcare practitioner to ensure that you're keeping everything in balance.

Alpha-Lipoic Acid

- "Universal" antioxidant that helps boost activity of vitamins C and E; made in the body
- Dosage: 200–800 mg a day

May be good for: Diabetes complications, and for boosting overall antioxidant activity in the body

Carotenoids

- Substances found in plants that appear to protect against various chronic diseases
- Dosage: 25 mg a day

May be good for: Aiding resistance to cancer and heart disease; studies show carotenoids can help prevent sunburn when taken regularly

Coenzyme Q$_{10}$

- Found in every body cell; essential for cellular metabolism
- Dosage: 50–200 mcg a day

May be good for: Prevention of heart disease, treatment of heart failure and hypertension, improving energy levels

Fiber

- Indigestible parts of plant foods with well-documented, health-promoting effects; can be taken as supplemental powders or tablets
- Dosage: 14 grams per 1,000 calories consumed; 50 years and younger: 38 grams a day for men, 25 grams a day for women; over 50: 30 grams a day for men, 21 grams a day for women

Flavonoids

- Also called bioflavonoids; 4,000 different ones synthesized by plants; abundant in nature, high in apples, citrus fruits, grape seeds, green tea, onions, red wine, soy
- Dosage: 500 mg a day (along with 1,000 mg a day of vitamin C)

May be good for: Aiding absorption of vitamin C; promising research suggests anti-cancer activity, cardiovascular support, blood-vessel strength, possibly helping to prevent or treat hemorrhoids and varicose veins; anti-inflammatory, anti-allergy effects; improving liver detoxification

Lutein

- A carotenoid found in leafy greens; kale and avocados are good sources
- Dosage: 6–20 mg a day

May be good for: Helping to prevent cataract and macular degeneration; may have protective effects against prostate cancer

Omega-3 Fatty Acids

- Found primarily in fish oils and flaxseeds, and chia seed

- Dosage: 600–1,000 mg a day of combined ALA, DHA, EPA

May be good for: Inflammation; large body of research suggests role of these fats in cancer prevention, heart disease, and skin disease—and as a natural therapy for ADHD, bipolar disorder, and depression

Remember that supplements are not a replacement for dark leafy greens, deeply colored berries, whole grains, garlic, onions, or any of the other food staples of a health-promoting, disease-preventive diet. Multivitamin/ mineral supplements aren't disease cures, but there is good evidence they help prevent disease by ensuring that our micronutrient bases are covered.

For more information and resources on nutritional supplements, turn to the resources section.

CHAPTER 3

HERBAL MEDICINE

Herbal medicine has a tradition that goes back a lot farther than you might think—to before the dawn of humankind. Many animals, including bears, chimpanzees, elephants, and monkeys, use specific plants for medicinal purposes. Mankind has long observed this in the animal kingdom and has used some of the same plants for similar purposes. Since before written history, plant-based medicines have been a mainstay of medical care all over the world.

Herbs
Any of various, often aromatic, seed-producing plants used in medicine or seasoning that do not develop woody tissue and die down at the end of the growing season.

Herbs were phased out of American medicine after the 1940s, as vaccines, antibiotics, and modern surgical techniques took the wind out of herbal medicine's sails. The timeless tradition of plant medicine—and the connection it once helped us maintain with the natural world—all but disappeared in the United States.

Still, there's hope. The World Health Organization estimates that some 4 billion people worldwide use some form of herbal medicine today. In China, Europe, India and Japan, herbal medicine is as highly respected as pharmaceutical-based medicine, and is often used alongside allopathic drugs.

Herbal Medicine
Study or use of medicinal herbs to treat conditions or promote health and healing. To date, only 10 percent of 260,000 herbs with healing potential have been studied.

Here, we introduce you to

a few herbs that have stood the test of time and garnered a stamp of approval from both the natural and allopathic medical worlds. We categorize the herbs based on the use for which there is the most scientific documentation, but, as you'll see, just about every herb is a switch-hitter that works to balance the body in many ways at once.

> If you are pregnant or nursing and wish to use herbs, consult an herbalist, midwife, lactation consultant, or physician trained in their use.

Herb Forms

We'll assume you are not planning to forage for herbs in the wild, or try to make your own herbal supplements. If you have time for that, terrific, but most people don't. Here are the most likely forms of herbs you will find when you go shopping:

Whole Herbs

In the case of some herbs, such as basil, garlic, ginger, or rosemary, you have the option of buying them in the market and using them in your cooking. Powdered and dried herbs are also considered whole, as, of course, are the products of your own herb garden.

Decoctions, Infusions, and Teas

Some herbs can be purchased loose as fresh or dried plant parts to be made into a tea or infusion (a very strong tea). A *decoction* is a very strong tea made with bark, roots, or tubers. Teas, decoctions, and infusions have been the primary form of herbal medicine since its beginnings.

Tinctures

Pure or diluted spirits, or alcohol, are used to extract an herb's medicinal properties. Tinctures make all of the herb's constituents available to the body—both the water- and oil-soluble varieties. The tinctures have a longer shelf life than capsules—about five years, compared to a year or so for capsules. Unfortunately, tinctures often taste awful, but mixing them with a little water or juice can help.

Capsules

These can vary dramatically in quality. Some contain dried, chopped-up plants, and others contain extracts that are standardized for a certain amount of the most active ingredients, or are otherwise altered to make them more bioavailable and effective.

As we recommend the various herbs, we'll try to offer guidelines on how to choose the best version. Keep in mind, however, that new products come out all the time. If you are at all concerned about whether you're getting the best herbal bang for your buck, consult with an herbalist or naturopathic doctor. You can also call the herb companies directly for information.

Herbs for Immunity

This type of medicinal herb supports the immune system and helps eliminate bacteria, fungi, viruses, yeasts, or other substances that can do harm to the body.

Garlic

This fragrant culinary herb is used around the world to lower cholesterol, prevent excessive blood stickiness, and enhance overall circulatory health. Many of its components appear to aid in cancer prevention and improve the liver's ability to rid the body of toxins. Garlic can zap bacterial, fungal, parasitic, and viral infections, including drug-resistant strains of *E. coli*, the fungus *Candida albicans*, and intestinal parasites, such as *Giardia lamblia*.

The whole bulb contains ingredients that interact with one another when it is crushed or chewed, producing the compounds that are believed to be most beneficial. If the smell of garlic bothers you or your loved ones, try an odorless garlic preparation. Studies show that AGE (aged garlic extract) is plenty effective when it comes to busting bacteria, fungi, and viruses—at least in a test tube.

Try to eat at least one clove of fresh garlic a day, raw or cooked—about one gram. Chewing it freshly crushed is best. If you choose a garlic supplement, use freeze-dried garlic standardized to 1.3 percent alliin or 0.6% allicin. Take 600–900 mg per day.

Echinacea and Others

Research has found that echinacea has anti-inflammatory, immune-activating, and wound-healing properties. Revered by Native American Indians, this plant medicine has become one of the most common herbs used today, especially for the common cold. Controversy over echinacea's effectiveness in preventing and/or beating back a cold may be due to formula variations and strengths of doses used: for example, whether liquid, tablets, or capsules were taken. Variations in study designs have also created widely varying results in studies of echinacea.

The most positive study results have come from well-established, high-quality products, such as EchinaGuard from Nature's Way or Echinamide from Natural Factors. Also consider Esberitox, a combination of echinaceas, white cedar, and wild indigo—a clinically proven German natural medicine, available from Enzymatic Therapy.

If you have a ragweed allergy, you may have a cross-sensitization to echinacea, and may be served better with another herbal remedy. Other impressive newcomers worth using to support immune and respiratory health include: 1) Umcka ColdCare, made from an African herb, which offers impressive support for the immune system's response to the common cold; 2) an American ginseng extract product called Cold-fX; and 3) *Andrographis paniculata*, a proven adaptogen with a long history of use in both TCM and Ayurveda.

These herbal offerings can help you recover

faster, with fewer and less intense symptoms, but may not prevent their onset. In general, begin to take the herbal remedy as soon as you start to feel the earliest symptoms of a cold or flu. It's best to take these remedies for five days to three weeks to knock out symptoms. Use for no more than six to eight weeks without taking a one to two week break, as they lose their effectiveness when taken long term.

Herbs for Inflammation

Hidden, chronic, slow-burning inflammation—an immune-system imbalance that creates chronic irritation within the body—has been linked with the diseases that debilitate and end the lives of too many people in first-world countries, including Alzheimer's disease, arthritis, cancer, and heart disease. Herbs with anti-inflammatory actions work by some of the same mechanisms as the popular anti-inflammatory drugs, but their mode of action is broader and gentler, and there is no evidence of the side effects that have led to warnings and recalls of those drugs.

Inflammation
Externally, an immune response to infection or injury that involves redness, swelling, and pain. Internally, silent chronic inflammation continuously assaults the body's defense systems.

Ginger

Ginger has a long history of use as a remedy for nausea and motion sickness. Ginger tea is a time-tested remedy for nasal congestion, coughs, and sore throat.

Ginger is a natural anti-inflammatory that inhibits the COX-1 and COX-2 enzymes, with COX-2 being the target of most non-narcotic pain and arthritis drugs. In one study of a group of people with osteo- or rheumatoid arthritis, more than three-quarters of them found significant relief in pain and swelling when they took a powdered ginger supplement.

Ginger extract inhibits the activation of genes

that spur inflammation in beta-amyloid, a substance found abundantly in brain tissue that is affected by Alzheimer's. In other experiments, two ginger phytochemicals, gingerol and paradol, slowed the formation of cancers in mice that had been exposed to environmental toxins.

Use grated or minced ginger in cooking. Make ginger tea by boiling slices of ginger root, one ounce per pint of water, for 20 to 30 minutes.

Turmeric

Ayurvedic medicine uses turmeric to treat colic, flatulence, inflammation, jaundice, and menstrual complaints. Turmeric is a powerful anti-inflammatory that is used in India as standard drug therapy for arthritis. It is one of nature's most effective antioxidants and has antimicrobial properties too. Other studies show that turmeric suppresses cancer initiation and metastasis (spread).

Add turmeric or curry powder to grains, meats, and rice. A marinade made with turmeric and garlic cuts down on the formation of carcinogenic chemicals formed during the grilling of meats. As a supplement, use capsules containing turmeric powder standardized to 95-percent curcumin. Follow dosage directions on the label.

> Anyone with breast cancer should talk to a nutritionally aware healthcare professional before using turmeric or curcumin supplements. The herb may interact negatively with drugs used to treat the disease.

Brain-Boosting, Circulation-Enhancing Herb—Ginkgo Biloba

Ginkgo biloba relaxes blood vessels, allowing more blood to flow through and into tissues and organs; it blocks platelet aggregation, the clumping together of platelets that thickens blood and slows its flow through the body. Together, these effects promote better circulation of oxygen- and nutrient-rich blood to the brain, heart, and extremities.

Ginkgo helps to improve verbal recall in people with mild age-related memory loss. It is an effective treatment for intermittent claudication, where blood vessels in the legs become painfully clogged; and it is a promising treatment for chronic ringing in the ears (tinnitus).

And it fights inflammation and neutralizes disease-promoting free radicals, a double whammy believed to greatly benefit people with Alzheimer's, cancer, heart disease, and rheumatoid arthritis. In healthy people, ginkgo may boost energy, improve well-being, and ease asthma symptoms.

Look for a standardized extract of ginkgo such as Ginkgold, made by Nature's Way. Ginkgold contains 60 mg of dried ginkgo biloba leaf extract, standardized to 24 percent flavone glycosides and 6 percent terpene lactones.

Adaptogenic and Immune-Enhancing Herbs

Adaptogenic herbs are herbs that help to balance and energize the body. Their effects help align the body toward balance, regardless of which direction it needs to go in order to get there. For example: if your immune system is underactive, adaptogens increase its activity; if you have an autoimmune condition, adaptogens tone down the immune response.

Adaptogens
Substances that increase resistance to biological, chemical, or physical stresses, and that aid the body in recovering from stress.

Eleuthero

Eleuthero is used to treat age-related memory loss, fatigue, female problems, headaches, impotence, low energy, and stomachaches. It is popular among athletes, astronauts, deep-sea divers, soldiers, and others with physically or mentally taxing occupations. It increases energy and the capacity to do work, while calming the nervous system. Eleuthero increases resistance against colds and flu.

Try 100–200 mg, two to three times per day, of a standardized extract in pill or tincture form. It's most effective when used long-term. Wild eleuthero is our favorite.

Panax Ginseng

This tonic adaptogenic herb increases the amount of oxygen that passes from the bloodstream into the cells to be burned for energy, thereby improving exercise performance and facilitating the breakdown of carbohydrate and fat stores. These effects explain why ginseng is so popular as an energy and endurance booster. It is also thought to increase the availability of glucose (fuel) in the brain, enhancing alertness and thinking ability.

During periods of stress, hormones released from the adrenal glands alter the body's chemistry in ways that increase alertness, dexterity, energy, and physical strength. Specific chemicals called ginsenosides have been found to behave much like those hormones, attaching to the same receptor sites and leading to some of the same physiological changes.

Ginseng is an antioxidant, and it also appears to improve the body's production of glutathione—an important natural antioxidant. Ginseng may forestall cancer by acting as an anti-inflammatory and antioxidant, and by suppressing growth of the new blood vessels required to feed tumors. Ginseng speeds healing from colds and flu, improves the effectiveness of a flu vaccination, and activates immunity during an infectious illness. And ginseng has long been used to heighten sexual desire, pleasure, and performance.

Try an extract of panax ginseng, the most-researched type, standardized to between 1.5 and 7 percent ginsenoside, at a dosage of 200–400 mg per day. It is most effective when taken over long periods, but take a two-week break from the herb every four to six weeks. People with hypertension, or anyone who uses insulin or oral hypoglycemic drugs for diabetes should not use ginseng without supervision.

Better Circulatory Health with Hawthorn

Hawthorn lowers blood pressure and improves the heart's pumping strength. It improves blood flow to the heart muscle, strengthens blood vessels, and may help keep blood from thickening and clotting too much. Rats given hawthorn before having a heart attack induced had less damage to the heart muscle compared with rats not given the herb.

In one study, there was significant improvement of fatigue, shortness of breath, and palpitations in people with heart failure who were taking hawthorn compared with a control group taking a placebo. Those on hawthorn used fewer medications for blood pressure and control of their heart rates.

Find a standardized extract containing 1.8 to 2.2 percent vitexin and use it according to the directions on the label. If you have heart disease or are taking any medications, let your medical team know you're using hawthorn.

Summing Up

In this overview, we have barely touched on the wide variety of herbs that are available and backed by historical, empirical use and scientific studies. Herbs can be used on their own or alongside mainstream medicine. Some herbs do have interactions with drugs, so if you are using any allopathic medications, check with your pharmacist and doctor before adding a new herb.

For more information and resources, turn to the resources section.

CHAPTER 4

HOMEOPATHY

Homeopathy was developed in the late 1700s by Samuel Hahnemann, a German physician, and was the subject of much investigation in the early part of the nineteenth century. Today, mainstream medicine is at odds with the theory behind homeopathy, claiming that it is based on junk science, and that any efficacy it might have is due to factors other than the remedies themselves. Alternative medical practitioners and millions of happy homeopathy users disagree.

The word *homeopathy* is derived from the Greek *homoios* (similar) and *pathos* (suffering). It is based on the principle of similars, where like cures like. Rather than suppressing disease, homeopathy uses substances that stimulate the natural process of healing. This isn't as far-fetched as it sounds at first. A fever is often best treated by bundling up so the fever breaks with a sweat. Vaccines stimulate natural immunity against diseases by exposing people (and animals) to killed viruses or bacteria (or pieces of them). Allergy shots work this way, too, putting small amounts of allergenic substances into the body to desensitize allergic reactions to them.

To make a homeopathic remedy, a substance is subjected to serial dilution, where several parts of water or alcohol are added, and then to succussion, a process where the mixture is subjected to high-energy shaking. These processes are repeated several times. Finally, small sugar pellets are saturated with the resulting solution, or it is used to make a liquid medicine.

Homeopathic medicines can look very much like conventional medicines, although they work in a

completely different way. They can be given in liquid, tablet, pellet, granule, cream, or spray forms.
Over 60 percent of homeopathic remedies are prepared from vegetable or plant materials. Others are
made from a wide variety of plant, animal, insect, or
mineral substances.

Homeopathic medicines are prepared by taking
the selected material and putting it through a metic-
ulous process of serial dilution and succussion (vig-
orous shaking), with dilution levels frequently going
beyond the level where any remnant of the original
substance can be detected. A remedy's potency
describes the measure of its dilution and is denoted
by the number that follows the name of the medicine itself, like Arnica 3x or 10c. The higher the number, the greater the dilution has occurred. The x
means it has been diluted by a factor of 10; the c
means it has been diluted by a factor of 100. According to homeopathic philosophy, the greater the
dilution, the more energetically powerful and deeper acting the resulting remedy.

Much of the controversy about homeopathy aris-
es from the belief that homeopathic remedies are
so diluted that no actual molecules of the original
substance are left. Even prominent homeopathic
physicians admit that no one really knows how it
works. But anyone who has successfully used homeopathic medicine—usually with the aid of a skilled
practitioner—will tell you it *does* work. And case
studies and research comparing homeopathy with
placebo treatments support its efficacy.

The Proof Is in the Proving?

The remedies used today were developed using
a process called *proving*. Hahnemann gathered
healthy subjects and administered doses of hun-
dreds of potential homeopathic remedies, including herbs, minerals, pharmaceuticals, even snake
venom or cuttlefish ink. The subjects' physical, emotional, and spiritual responses to those substances
were carefully catalogued. Based on those respons-

es, Hahnemann figured out which of those substances—in greatly diluted form—could be applied to various ailments with those symptoms experienced to restore balance and health.

Since then, there have been many placebo-controlled repeats of Hahnemann's method of proving, and his reasoning was sound. The remedies' effects on healthy people are an accurate indication of which symptoms they should be used to treat.

Some Theories About How Homeopathy Works

Hahnemann and those who follow in his footsteps believe that the combination of dilution and succussion creates a new kind of substance, an energetic imprinting of the original ingredient. The remedy conveys information to the body about what and how to heal. Although it defies scientific explanation, we know that homeopathic remedies don't only work through a placebo effect. They work in people who are unconscious, in infants, and in animals. Placebo-controlled studies show consistent differences between responses to homeopathics and placebos.

Placebo Effect
Where an inactive substance, usually a sugar pill, has healing effects—probably because of the person's belief that the medicine will help them heal.

Chemists and physicists are finding that the liquid in which the herbs, minerals, or other substances are succussed actually changes on a molecular level, maintaining some kind of an imprint of the original substance. One group of Italian chemists has found changes in the electrical conductivity of homeopathic solutions diluted and succussed from 3C to 30C that could help explain why homeopathic remedies—which these chemists call "medicine without molecules"—seem to work such magic.

The likely truth is that no clinical trial or laboratory experiment involving homeopathic medicines will ever satisfy skeptics. The process of homeopathic treatment involves more than taking medicines; the detailed consultations between the caregiver and the person being treated probably play a significant role in the healing process.

Homeopathy doesn't require any kind of diagnosis. Treatment is based on a detailed evaluation of symptoms, and remedies are applied based on those symptoms, rather than on a diagnosis of underlying disease. This circumvents the problems of misdiagnosis, false diagnosis, and difficult diagnosis that are often encountered in allopathic medicine. It also circumvents the tendency of allopathy to create new diseases, disorders, or syndromes to justify drug treatment.

Research That Supports the Effectiveness of Homeopathic Medicine

All this said, there is a considerable body of research that supports the effectiveness of homeopathic remedies for the treatment of common health problems. Here is a sampling.

- A study by French researchers at Boiron, a company that makes homeopathic remedies, found that 499 children (aged eighteen months to four years) with recurrent colds had significantly fewer colds in a six-month period when they used homeopathic remedies (2.71 bouts of colds vs. 3.97 bouts).

- A German study compared a homeopathic remedy, Gripp-Heel, to conventional treatment for mild viral infections (with symptoms like coughing, fever, headache, muscle pain, or sore throat) in 485 people. At the study's end, 67.9 percent of those using homeopathy no longer had symptoms, while only 47.9 of those on conventional treatments were without symptoms at that point. A lack of side effects and the ease of treatment was rated at 88.9 percent by those using homeopathic remedies compared to 38.8 percent in the conventional treatment group.

- Several studies have found that the cold and flu remedy oscillococcinum speeds recovery and reduces symptom severity.

- A German study found that the homeopathic nasal spray Luffa comp.-Heel worked as well as the drug cromolyn sodium to relieve symptoms of hay fever.

- A series of British studies found that individually prescribed homeopathic remedies improved breathing test scores and respiratory function in people with asthma.

For every one of the positive studies published in medical journals, there are many more stories of healing told by practitioners and people who have been helped. Homeopathy has little potential for harm. Even a small child can swallow a whole bottle of homeopathic tablets without danger.

What to Expect from a Homeopathic Practitioner

A homeopath knows that two people presenting with the same health problem—let's say a cold—may require very different remedies to draw them back into a balanced state.

When you go to see a homeopath, expect to answer a lot of questions. She or he will talk with you about genetic, behavioral, and lifestyle issues, as well as physical symptoms of disease, to develop a complete picture of you, the person being treated. Then, the homeopath will make an individualized prescription, and will make remedies for you or tell you where to buy them. They may be in the form of small pellets to be dissolved under the tongue, sprays, liquids, or ointments. He or she will follow your course as you use the remedies, and will probably have you back for at least one follow-up. Once you have learned how the process works, and about how your particular personality interplays with your symptoms, you will be able to self-treat with confidence for minor or self-limiting health problems.

For more information and resources, turn to the resources section.

CHAPTER 5

MANIPULATIVE THERAPIES— CHIROPRACTIC AND OSTEOPATHIC

Manipulative therapies, often called *physical medicine*, can refer to any of the many therapies that involve physical manipulation of the body. Manipulative therapies have been practiced since ancient times in Egypt, Greece, and China. In this chapter, we'll focus on two well-established fields: chiropractic and osteopathy.

Chiropractic

Modern chiropractic was officially founded in North America by Daniel Palmer in 1895. Today's doctor of chiropractic is a primary-care physician who specializes in natural, non-surgical, and drugless therapies, with a focus on manual treatments. The term *chiropractic* is derived from the Greek for "done with the hands"—specifically, medical care through manipulation or adjusting, with a special emphasis on care and correction of the spine. Chiropractors receive extensive training at accredited chiropractic colleges, and are licensable in all fifty states.

Chiropractors diagnose and treat people whose health problems are associated mostly with the body's musculoskeletal and nervous systems. The entire spine is of special importance; most of the connective interactions of our nerves and blood vessels start in the spine and extend from there to all other parts of the body.

By correcting problems with posture and body mechanics, and by freeing up subluxations—joints that are stuck out of place from injury, tension, or other factors—chiropractors restore full range of motion to the body. The resulting improvements go well beyond the areas of the body that have been worked on, although immediate pain relief and normalized function are often experienced in the office. Improved energy; less overall pain; better balance; greater flexiblility and strength; reduced numbness and tingling in hands, feet, shoulders, neck, and head; headache relief; and relief from low back pain, sciatica, other types of limb neuropathies, and carpal tunnel syndrome have all been reported with chiropractic treatment.

The chiropractic healthcare system is based, essentially, on a simple and profound premise: *structure dictates function.* If the body's structure is compromised, then health will be negatively impacted. The structure and alignment of the spinal column have special importance in the function of the body, because of the spine's relationship to the transmission of nerve impulses to and from the cord. If there is a problem with nerve transmission, expression, or communication within the body, there will be a corresponding problem, limitation, dysfunction, and/or pain related to the affected nerves and structures involved.

By correcting the structural problems that are causing the discomfort—usually in the spine, joints, and related connective tissues—it is possible to recover and return to healthy, pain-free functioning.

At a visit to a chiropractor, you will be asked about your overall health, lifestyle, diet, and work and family life, thereby providing the doctor with the information needed to gain a deep understanding of the root of your health problem. The examination will vary, depending upon your chiropractor's specific techniques, but will often include muscle testing, kinesiology, range-of-motion testing, postural analysis, and analysis of structural abnormalities from surgery, stress, or injury. Blood work may be ordered, and x-rays may be part of a more indepth consultation when indicated.

The chiropractor may then use his or her hands to precisely manipulate and adjust joints and parts of the spine, with the goal of stimulating healing, improving flow of nerve energy, blood, and lymph fluid. These manipulations aim to normalize and restore full mobility and function. (There is a difference between *manipulation* and *adjusting*, but for our purposes, these terms are interchangeable.)

An adjustment is generally a high-velocity, low-amplitude thrusting movement performed on or at a joint or joints, often accompanied by a popping or clunking sound. While dramatic, it is harmless and natural. From an observer's viewpoint, it may look and sound horrible, but from the recipient's side, it is the opposite: although it may occasionally cause a brief moment of pain, any pain from a correctly performed chiropractic adjustment quickly gives way to pleasurable release of tension and relief from pain, along with renewed strength and vitality.

In general, you can expect to feel improvements in your musculoskeletal problems in one to five sessions. Keep in mind, however, that everybody is different, and not all chiropractors practice alike. Ask them after your initial consultation and examination what kind of treatment they suggest, and what you might reasonably expect in terms of improvement. You can't expect miracles, but you can expect legitimate improvement in many conditions in a reasonably short period of time. If you don't get it, seek another practitioner. In general, a 25 to 80 percent improvement can been seen with chiropractic treatment in as little as a week to up to a month, depending on the condition.

The Importance of Correct Diagnosis

With any medical condition, be careful to obtain a correct diagnosis before entering into any treatment. If it takes a second or even a third opinion from a variety of practitioners, ensure that you don't miss a serious ailment that could have been treated successfully early on if it hadn't been ignored. In the end, you are responsible for your health and your healthcare decisions. Certain tumors or disease processes can start out as diffuse aches, pains, or minor-seeming complaints. While manipulation may bring some relief, the underlying condition may continue to develop.

In choosing a chiropractor—or any healthcare provider—get a personal referral whenever possible. Choose someone who instills trust and is caring, honest, professional, and dedicated to his or her career. Avoid practitioners who rush patients in and out with quick and frequent visits. We suggest that you find a doctor of chiropractic who takes the time needed, with joy, and listens to both your spoken needs and your body's unspoken ones.

Osteopathy

A doctor of osteopathy is a licensed primary-care doctor who has equal status to an M.D. There are twenty-two accredited osteopathic medical schools, and osteopaths can be licensed in all fifty states. In the United States, there are currently an estimated 44,000 practicing osteopaths.

Their scope of practice is legally identical to the medical mainstream—they can work in hospitals, practice surgery, and prescribe drugs—but they have a different philosophical heritage. Today, many D.O.s practice exactly like M.D.s, in a less than holistic fashion; others choose to stay close to their origins and practice manipulation, nutritional therapeutics, and other natural therapies.

Like chiropractors, osteopaths have specialized training in anatomy and physiology, with focus on the body's structural elements and biomechanics. Osteopathy's underlying belief is that physical structure affects our functioning. "Special education" for muscles, nerves, and bones is an important aspect of this medical philosophy, as the interplay of these systems strongly impacts health and disease.

Our bodies know how to heal when obstacles are removed and the opportunity to heal is created and supported. This is a central theme for physical medicine specifically and for natural medicine in general. Healing occurs when life force is flowing freely and able to bring its healing energies wherever they are needed. Osteopathy, in concept, attempts to correct imbalances in our structural system, enabling the body to rebalance and self-heal.

The osteopathic concept of disease and healing centers on the supreme adaptability of the human body, within and out. For example, just by shifting your weight from two feet to one foot, a complex series of changes instantly occurs within your muscular and skeletal systems from head to toe, allowing you to reestablish balance and equilibrium in your new position. A similar process occurs in response to injury or stresses. If the injury does not resolve spontaneously, but persists, then various adaptations in other parts of the body are made and persist. Structural changes and changes in circulation and nerve impulses produce areas of greater susceptibility to infection, pain, dysfunction, or degeneration. The whole range of these subsequent changes makes up the diverse array of disease.

Osteopaths use a system of manipulation that differs from that of chiropractors. Osteopathic manipulative technique (OMT) involves stretching, gentle pressure, and muscular resistance from the recipient to move muscles and joints. With the recipient sitting or lying down on a table, a doctor of osteopathy gently applies a precise amount of manual pressure in a specific direction, either to put the tissues at ease or to engage them at their functional limit. The D.O. may also use techniques similar to the "thrusting" style of chiropractic adjustment.

OMT aims to treat structural and tissue abnormalities (vertebrae, muscles, connective tissues); relieve joint restriction and misalignment; restore muscle and tissue balance; promote circulation; improve joint range of motion; and balance tissue and muscle mechanics.

For information on finding a chiropractor or osteopath, turn to the resources section.

CHAPTER 6

MASSAGE THERAPIES AND BODYWORK

Touch is as vital to human health as healthy food and pure water. Babies and children who are not adequately touched are stunted both physically and emotionally. During childhood, our nervous systems develop largely in response to touch. And few would argue that we do not need tender, loving touch in adulthood and later life.

A good bodyworker—a practitioner of massage or other hands-on healing therapies—can reeducate a body that has lost its native intelligence from sitting too often and not exercising enough. She or he can move energy around in the body to help it heal, or free up areas of the body that have become constricted, stiff, or painful.

Bodywork can increase coordination, flexibility, and physical intelligence—the body's accurate responsiveness to the needs of our lives. It can improve immunity and help lift depression. It can release us from postural or movement habits that are causing the body to degenerate and hurt. And, finally, most bodywork just *feels good.*

Bodywork has been found to effectively move fluids—blood and the lymph between organs—around in the body. By releasing constrictions in connective tissue and muscle, and by moving tissues around, bodywork promotes the circulation of fresh, oxygenated, nutrient-rich blood and immune-cell-filled lymph. It can aid in balancing gland function.

Deane Juhan, who practices his bodywork art at the Esalen Institute in Big Sur, California, writes that ". . . the bodyworker is not an interventionist; he is a facilitator, a diplomatic intermediary between physiological processes that have lost track of one another's proper functions and goals . . . Touching hands are not like pharmaceuticals or scalpels. They are like flashlights in a darkened room. The medicine they administer is self-awareness. And for many of our painful conditions, this is the aid that is most urgently needed."

Types of Bodywork

Regardless what form of bodywork you choose, the ultimate goal is to know yourself better and to evolve into a more relaxed and healthy version of that self. You can feel confident that no matter which methods you choose (you can choose more than one), if you go into it with an attitude of openness and curiosity, it will facilitate your path toward healing. Bodywork can be done clothed, partially clothed, or without clothes; the level of undress depends on the type of work being done. Talk with the practitioner about what's expected and, if necessary, discuss your comfort level.

Aromatherapy Massage

This type of massage combines aromatherapy and Swedish massage (see page 52), using oils scented with plant and flower essences to address specific health issues during the massage.

Chair Massage

Chair massage is done fully clothed in a special chair in which the recipient leans forward and the upper body is worked on. Sometimes called *corporate massage.*

Deep Tissue Massage

This type of massage is commonly used after an injury, when damage to ligaments, muscles, or tendons has resulted in contracted areas around joints. The therapist uses deep pressure and slow strokes across and with the grain of muscles, tendons, and *fascia* (the tough connective tissue that surrounds muscles and tendons).

Infant Massage

As taught today, infant massage has proven to be good medicine for chest and sinus congestion, colic, release of emotional stress, and teething. Infant massage improves a baby's digestive function, enhances the development of the nervous system, and makes the baby sleep better. Massage is particularly beneficial for premature babies. You can bring your infant to specially trained practitioners or learn to do infant massage on your own from books, classes, DVDs, and videos.

Lymphatic Massage

This involves gentle, light massaging along the lymph channels and over the lymph nodes to aid in excess fluid retention (edema) and the removal of toxins. It is believed to help relieve chronic sinusitis and post-surgical swelling, and some find it helps ease their arthritis.

Neuromuscular Therapy/Myotherapy

Also known as Trigger Point Therapy, this type of massage utilizes finger pressure against specific trigger points that are often tender and painful. It is helpful for breaking cycles of pain and spasm that establish themselves in the body following illness, injury, or stress.

Pregnancy Massage

Massages can be very helpful for pregnant women, but they should be massaged only by therapists with certifications in prenatal massage.

Rolfing

This is short for Rolfing Structural Integration, a bodywork method developed by Ida P. Rolf. She was seeking to create methods for working on deep myofascial structures in order to release adhesions and tensions that restricted free motion. Rolfing is based on the belief that, left unresolved, those tensions and adhesions impede the body's ability to organize itself into a state of optimal health and well-being. Although many people swear by Rolfing, and it has stood the test of time as an effective form of bodywork, you should know one thing up front—it hurts. But those who endure the requisite series of ten treatments say it's worth it for the relief that follows the treatments.

Any true Rolfer can document going through the proper training based on Ida Rolf's techniques. Visit www.rolf.org for more information and certification guidelines, or call 1-303-449-5903, ext. 100, to find a Rolfer in your area.

Shiatsu

This combination of pressure and assisted stretching draws on techniques used in acupressure, massages, including lymphatic massage (which focuses on moving lymph through the lymph vessels), osteopathy, and physical therapy. It is performed with the fully dressed client on a padded floor. Unlike acupressure, with which it is often confused, shiatsu applies pressure over wider areas than acupressure points, and the therapist's elbows, feet, knees, and palms may be involved in the massage. The shiatsu therapist applies gradual rhythmic pressure along the meridians (energy channels) and may engage in something that feels like a laying on of hands. In addition to stretching, manipulative techniques and a wide variety of touches, including brushing, pinching, plucking, rotating, shaking, and vibrating, may be integrated. Go to www.aobta.org, the website of the American Organization for Body Work Therapies of Asia, which accredits schools and teachers. Click on Member Database to find a shiatsu practitioner near you.

Sports Massage

Designed specifically for athletes to help keep them flexible and protect against injury. This type of massage has also become popular with non-athletes.

Swedish Massage

This is the most common form of massage. It employs various strokes, such as *effleurage* (smooth, gliding strokes to relax soft tissues), *petrissage* (kneading, squeezing, and rolling muscles between the fingers), *tapotement* (where cupped hands, fingers, or the edges of hands are used in short alternating taps), and *friction* (deeper circular movements that rub layers of tissue against one another, increasing blood flow to the area). Swedish massage therapists may move body parts around in their natural range of motion to release tension and lightly stretch the muscles.

Thai Massage

A synthesis of acupressure, assisted yoga poses and stretching, and shiatsu, this practice has been called yoga for the lazy. The client lies on the floor, fully dressed, and is manipulated into various positions by the therapist, who works along the meridians (energy channels) of the body that have been established in Chinese medicine. Starting at the feet and ending at the head, the therapist uses healing touch to foster better circulation of energy throughout the body, which can improve flexibility and loosen tight areas. Extensive training enables the therapist to effortlessly move the client around during the one- to three-hour treatment. Thai massage is done in silence.

> With the exception of Thai massage, there may be some conversation between massage therapist and client during the session. If you prefer silence during your massage, let the therapist know before you begin.

Beyond certification, be sure to find a massage therapist or bodyworker with whom you feel comfortable and relaxed. Feel free to tell the therapist what you want from the session. Avoid eating just before massage, and make sure you let the therapist know of any physical problems you are experiencing. Be communicative during the massage (only when necessary), too, reporting any excessive discomfort or problems with the environment—for example, if the music is too loud or distracting, or they are burning incense that irritates your nose.

Stay in touch with your breath throughout the massage. Allow yourself to breathe deeply, especially when the therapist is working in a tender or tense area. Let the therapist know if you are having trouble getting or staying relaxed.

Don't try to rush right back into a busy day after having bodywork done. Take time to relax and drink plenty of water. If the cost of bodywork is an issue, check with your local massage and bodywork schools to see whether they offer reduced-price or free sessions with their students.

For information on finding a qualified bodyworker or massage therapist, see the resources section.

CHAPTER 7

MIND/BODY THERAPIES

The idea of the mind and body as separate entities is a new one in the broad scale of history. After roughly two centuries of belief in the separation of the emotional, spiritual, and psychological from the physical and biochemical, the world has come back home to the same beliefs put forth by the ancients—that mind and body are integrated.

Mind/body medicine is a wonderfully integrative area of research that is bringing together the mainstream and natural medicine fields. Research abounds on the subject of how thoughts and feelings affect health and our responses to disease treatment. New scientific disciplines have emerged that show how genes and the inner workings of the body reflect the mind. And these, in turn, show how thoughts can be used to improve health and longevity, and how counseling, life coaching, meditation, prayer, qigong, spirituality, the arts, yoga, and regular doses of humor can help everyone live, not just healthier and longer, but also *happier* lives.

Spirituality

Being spiritual means you search for meaning and purpose in your day-to-day life, connecting with others, and moving beyond self-absorption. In the end, the spiritual quest is about finding a sense of inner peace and well-being that helps you appreciate each day, each moment, as a gift—even when things go wrong. Spirituality grounds you in the current moment and helps you see what is really important.

The spiritual life is characterized by study and

reflection, and the belief that all things are interconnected. Spirituality is often about *finding* more connection—with other people, with yourself, with the natural world, or with your ancestors.

Religion—a set of beliefs and practices that are usually culturally determined—aids in spirituality, giving seekers a path that many others travel and have traveled. Community and social support are often important aspects of religion, and both of these have powerful health-promoting effects aside from spirituality. But you don't have to be religious to be spiritual. Some people don't follow any specific discipline, but forge their own paths, finding their own ways to live spiritually based lives.

Whether religious or not, people who embrace spirituality are generally healthier and longer-lived, and enjoy a greater quality of life, though research suggests that involvement in religion has slightly more beneficial effects on lifespan. The social integration and sense of community and support offered by organized religion probably enhance the effects of spiritual living.

Spirituality and religion help both sick and well people enjoy a better quality of life. In one study, researchers gathered 216 chronically ill inpatients at a Midwestern hospital, including amputees and people with breast cancer, prostate cancer, post-polio syndrome, and spinal cord injury. Based on their responses to several questionnaires, the researchers divided the subjects into three groups: religious, existential (spiritual but not religious), and non-spiritual. Not surprisingly, the third group had a significantly lower quality of life and life satisfaction than the other two.

In traditional Asian medicine, it is believed that anxiety, tension, and unhappiness predispose people to cancer. It would follow that maintaining peace through spirituality would be protective, and the research suggests this is true. Although it is not yet known whether being spiritual can improve the chances of recovering from cancer, it is known that being spiritual improves the quality of life and the outlook of those with the disease, regardless of their prognosis.

Research shows that spiritual observances, psychotherapy, and psychosocial support decrease the risk of both depression and heart attacks in older people who have recently lost a spouse. Anxiety and depression are less common and more easily treated in people with religious or spiritual beliefs. And the medical community is finding that when they address these beliefs with those in their care, it improves the doctor/patient relationship and their patient's ability to move toward healing—or, if a person is terminally or incurably ill, toward a better quality of life.

Even if you have had a bad experience with organized religion, or you are skeptical about spirituality, there is a spiritual path that will work for you. If you are a firm believer in modern science and skeptical about spirituality, keep in mind that the greatest scientists of our time—Albert Einstein, for example—have been spiritual people. Einstein understood that our knowledge of the material world is dwarfed by what is not known, and he reveled in the part of science that is about mystery and questioning.

In the rest of this chapter, you'll find some ideas about how to enrich your spiritual life—and improve your health and well-being in the process.

Prayer

Prayer is a way of speaking to a higher power, of voicing our thoughts, feelings, needs, and problems in an atmosphere of safety. Science suggests that prayer is a powerful form of medicine that relieves anxiety and depression. Research on *distant intentionality*—the ability of focused prayer to alter the body functions of a person far away—suggests we may be able to support the health of others through prayer as well.

Prayer and Meditation
Prayer is when you talk to God;
Meditation is when you listen to God.
—Diana Robinson

Try returning to some of the prayers you learned as a child, or learn some new ones from your minister, priest, rabbi, or other religious teacher. The spirituality section of your bookstore will offer more alternatives. If you want to pray but don't know any prayers, create your own—just speak your mind from the heart.

Meditation

Meditation benefits a wide range of health conditions, including anxiety, depression, drug addiction, fibromyalgia, heart disease, high blood pressure, insomnia, irritable bowel syndrome, pain, premenstrual syndrome, stress-related illness, and tension headaches.

Transcendental Meditation (TM)

Transcentental meditation is a specific form of meditation that may prolong life expectancy. In the past twenty-five years, over 500 research studies have been conducted into TM and it's clear from these studies that TM is highly beneficial to mind and body.

All forms of transcendental meditation can be divided into two categories: *concentrative* and *mindfulness*. In concentrative meditation, you focus your attention on something—your breathing, a sound, or a visual image, for example. Yogic meditation tends to be concentrative, focusing on the meditator's own breath or chanting (mantras). Mindfulness meditation is more characteristic of Taoist and Zen practices. It involves sitting quietly and allowing thoughts to pass through the mind, just observing them and not reacting to them.

All meditation allows you to decrease the levels of stress hormones, lower your blood pressure and heart rate, and relax your body. Experienced meditators learn to enter a state of relaxed alertness, where the mind is wide awake and clear while the body is resting.

Try this: sit comfortably upright in a chair or on the floor. Close your eyes, turn your palms up in your lap, and breathe deeply, letting your abdomen expand, your shoulders drop and spread, and your sternum lift as you inhale. Let thoughts come and go, but don't react to, or act upon them. If you feel the need to concentrate your attention in order to become more relaxed, try counting backward from 100, with one count per exhalation.

Enlightened Exercise—Yoga and Qigong

The word yoga means *union* or *yoke*—joining together the body, mind, and soul. If your mental image of yoga simply involves beautiful people stretching their bodies into painful-looking positions, it's time to look at it differently. The study and practice of yoga is meant to calm the mind, reduce physical stress, and rejuvenate the body.

Yoga practice helps you prepare for the quiet of meditation. Some of the poses promote better digestive and endocrine (gland) function; others are designed to improve the body's ability to cleanse itself of toxins. It helps move vital energy—*prana* in Ayurveda, *qi* in traditional Asian medicine—around in the body. Yogic breathing—an essential part of yoga practice—is relaxing and invigorating, and can improve symptoms in people with asthma. Regular yoga practice improves cardiovascular health and a Harvard study has shown it to be an effective treatment for insomnia.

In traditional Chinese medicine (TCM), it is believed that with focused meditation, it is even possible to alter your own blood circulation. By directing your energy through qigong, you can foster an improved circulation of both energy and blood throughout your body.

The practice of qigong promotes greater sensitivity to the movement of qi within the body, and helps the practitioner direct it. It is believed that a qigong master can also emit qi to help others in their healing process. A study from the Center for Immunology at the University of Texas Southwestern Medical Center found that qigong practice enhanced the practitioners' immunity, reduced inflammation, slowed cellular metabolism, and even enhanced the expression of cancer-fighting genes.

The Arts—Dance, Music, Visual Arts, and Writing

In today's world, most people think of art as something to be done only by those who have talent or special training. But every person can benefit from expressing their emotions and thoughts through art. Dance, music, and art therapy are common forms of healing for exactly this reason. They help you open your heart and clear your mind.

Even if you've never danced a step, painted a picture, played an instrument, or written a poem, it isn't too late to start. Throughout history and cultures, art has been something for everyone—it isn't about being good at it, it's about the experience of creation and the way it makes you feel. And it's about continuing to learn new things throughout your life, a practice that keeps you young. Studies show there is a decrease in the risk for Alzheimer's and other forms of age-related memory loss when you keep your mind stimulated by learning new things.

Counseling and Life Coaching

Researchers in mind/body medicine have shown unequivocally that people's thought patterns have enormous sway over the functioning of their bodies. The question remains: how should thoughts be altered in order to improve health? Here are a few suggestions:

Cognitive-Behavioral Therapy (CBT)

This form of counseling is as effective as antidepressants for the treatment of anxiety and depression—both common problems in chronically ill people. CBT focuses on changing thought patterns in ways that foster an optimistic, relaxed, and constructive attitude toward life and relationships. Instead of unearthing old memories and trying to piece together *why* the person is feeling rotten, the CBT therapist focuses on the *now*, and on what can be changed today to improve the person's overall functioning and well-being. CBT usually involves only a short course of therapy, and is based on a treatment plan developed early on in the process. You can expect it to be a bit like school, with the therapist as teacher—there will even be homework.

Life Coaching

An athletic coach helps an athlete excel at his or her sport; a life coach can help you excel at *your life*. You can hire a specially trained coach to help you challenge your fears, identify the sources of your problems, and generally overcome life's obstacles. The coach is a confidante you can bounce ideas off and talk to as much as you like—an impartial helper who can focus all of her or his energy on helping you meet your goals. It can be costly—a few hundred dollars for a few coaching sessions—but it's an investment in yourself.

Humor

In his book *Anatomy of an Illness*, the journalist Norman Cousins wrote about being struck down with *ankylosing spondylitis*, a painful inflammatory condition. Doctors believed he might not survive, but they underestimated his determination to get better. He eschewed drugs, and developed his own treatment plan that involved megadoses of intravenous vitamin C and plenty of laughter. He holed up in a hotel room with a stack of funny movies—and he did get better.

It is widely known that laughter is healing. Finally waking up to this, the medical world has begun to publish research on the ways in which humor alters human immune function and other aspects of biochemistry. When feeling at your worst, turn on a funny movie or read a funny book. Visit your funniest friend. Seek out laughter on a daily basis, and make a point of indulging in at least one big boisterous laugh every day.

Return to the Moment

Here's one more small step you can take toward a more spiritual life that can make a huge difference. Anytime you are beginning to feel stressed or out of balance, return to the moment. Bring yourself unflinchingly into the now. Observe what's around you and be grateful for all you have. Find beauty wherever you are.

By choosing to read this book, you have expressed a commitment to maintaining optimal health. This kind of health is about enjoying your life, about feeling energetic and strong and loving. You can feel this way without a spiritual practice when things are going well, but when things go wrong, you may not have enough resources to fall back on without it.

For more information on mind/body work, turn to the resources section.

CHAPTER 8

AYURVEDIC MEDICINE

The word *Ayurveda* is made up of two Sanskrit words: *ayur*, meaning life, and *veda*, which means science. Unlike most other forms of medicine, Ayurvedic medicine is inseparable from its spiritual roots in Buddhism, Hinduism, and yoga. It views health as a balanced interplay between body, mind, and soul.

In Ayurvedic medicine, optimism, positivity, and a relaxed, balanced attitude are believed to foster recovery from illness. Too-hot passions are thought to predispose people to illness, and these beliefs mirror current knowledge about the potent effects of attitude and emotions on physical health.

Prakruti—Your Unique Constitution

One of Ayurvedic medicine's most basic tenets is that you are born with a constitution—a personality, a type, which was decided at the moment of your conception. This constitution, or *prakruti,* is fixed and unchangeable—reflecting all the current research on the importance of an individual's genetic make-up (determined at the moment of conception) to the individual they end up becoming.

According to Ayurveda, each person's constitution is made up of three *doshas,* or body-mind types. All three, *kapha, pitta,* and *vata,* are contained within every person, but in varying combinations.

Kapha

This dosha is believed to govern the structural aspects of the body—the bones, fluids, and sinews that give it shape and flexibility. Kapha-predominant people have lots of endurance and are even-tempered and calm. They tend to gain weight and are prone to lethargy (both mental and physical), procrastination, and sinus problems.

Pitta

This dosha is believed to govern digestion, hormone action, and metabolism—any body process that involves heat. Pitta-predominant people have fiery, intense dispositions and sharp minds, and tend toward angry, frustrated, or irritable responses to adversity. A hot temper and a reddish or flushed complexion has pitta written all over it. Typical illnesses for pitta-predominant individuals are heartburn, high blood pressure, skin rashes, and ulcers.

Vata

Lightness and movement are vata characteristics. If you are creative, enthusiastic, quick, talkative, thin, and tend towards anxiety, constipation, dry flaky skin, or intestinal gas, you are vata-dominant.

Ayurveda teaches that dietary and lifestyle choices running counter to your doshic constitution cause illness. Diet, herbs, internal cleansing, lifestyle changes, massage and other physical therapies, right thinking, and yoga, plus other types of breath work and exercise, are used to restore balance to the doshas. It's an elegantly simple system of healing that, similar to most natural medicine practices, focuses on maintaining optimal health rather than on rescuing the ill.

Visiting an Ayurvedic Doctor

A typical doctor's visit ranges from forty-five to ninety minutes in length. You will be asked many questions about your food preferences, your mental and physical attributes, and your personal and family history as the doctor determines your doshic profile. The doctor will listen to your heart and lungs and will examine your tongue. You may be asked to give a urine sample for analysis.

Measurements of the three superficial and three deep pulses are used to diagnose ailments of different organs. The tongue's color, coating, and sensitivity are used to help prescribe appropriate treatments. Often, the treatment plan includes herbs, including the following.

Amalaki

This herb builds and maintains new tissues, strengthens bones and teeth, and increases the red-blood-cell count. It reduces excessive pitta characteristics and is one of three herbs used in the tonic herbal combination *triphala.* Amalaki has been researched as a treatment for upset stomach.

Arjuna

Arjuna supports circulation and brings more oxygen to tissues. Ayurveda uses it to treat heart conditions, as it lowers both blood pressure and heart rate. It may be combined with other herbs (ashwagandha, brahmi, and guggul) in herbal formulas for heart health. Current research is also revealing an anti-cancer potential for this herb.

Ashwagandha

This is an adaptogenic, balancing herb that relieves exhaustion and general debility. It supports hormonal function, tissue healing, sleep quality, and better sexual function. It is being studied for its anti-cancer potential.

Bacopa (Brahmi)

This herb improves mental function and relaxes the body. It may be an effective aid for entering a state of relaxed focus, as for example, studying for, or taking, an exam.

Bibitaki

This is a laxative herb. It is the second part of the combination tonic triphala and it reduces excess kapha.

Bitter Melon

This is used to control blood sugar and insulin levels. It is effective in reducing cravings for sweets.

Boswellia

This is Ayurveda's herbal treatment for arthritis. It modulates immunity in ways that help reduce joint inflammation and pain. Research into its anti-inflammatory effects shows boswellia to be a promising herbal therapy for autoimmune and allergic diseases, such as asthma, colitis, Crohn's disease, and rheumatoid arthritis.

Guggul

This ancient treatment is used for infection and to decrease inflammation; more recently, research has shown it to be very effective for lowering elevated blood cholesterol.

Gymnema Sylvestre

This is another effective Ayurvedic remedy for balancing blood-sugar levels and reducing sugar cravings.

Haritaki

This herb, the third component of the triphala mixture, is used to treat asthma and coughs and is said to be especially good for vata types. One animal study found that it reduced the risk of cholesterol-induced heart disease.

Holy Basil

This is a popular supportive herb, used to promote better respiratory health.

Neem

Neem is one of the best-known Ayurvedic herbs, and virtually every part of this plant has a medicinal use. It has disinfectant and skin-healing qualities, is used to treat joint and muscle pain, and is widely used for dental care in India. Studies have revealed it to have antibacterial, anticarcinogenic, antifungal, antihyperglycemic, anti-inflammatory, antimalarial, antimutagenic, antioxidant, anti-ulcer, antiviral, and immune-boosting, properties.

Herbal Combinations

Formulations for common chronic conditions combine medicinal and culinary herbs. For example, the combination formula *chandraprabha* addresses both blood sugar and cholesterol and aids in weight control. *Hingvastak* reduces flatulence and bloating, and supports digestion. A well-known herbal combination for joint health (Artrex, also sold as Joint Formula) contains ashwaghanda, boswellia, ginger, and turmeric. *Shilagit* is a combination of herbs used to improve prostate health and promote the health of the urinary tract. *Trikatu*, a combination of black pepper, ginger, and pippali, is a digestive tonic and internal cleanser. *Triphala*, the popular herb combination of amalaki, bibitaki, and haritaki, is used to promote better digestion and blood oxygenation and the loss of excess fat. It is commonly taken over extended periods by people of all doshic types. *Liv.52* (LiverCare), which contains arjuna, black nightshade, capers, chicory, negro coffee, tamarisk, and yarrow, improves liver enzyme function, enhancing its ability to cleanse the body of toxins. LiverCare is supported by strong clinical research studies.

> Some Ayurvedic herbal remedies have been found to contain toxic levels of heavy metals. Buy herbs from a reputable source to assure that they are free of toxins.

Meditation in Ayurveda

Contrary to popular belief, meditation does not require that you sit motionless for hours with a completely empty mind, chanting mantras to attain enlightenment. In the West, meditation is commonly believed to require complete stillness and serenity. But some forms of meditation are waking and moving—think of the whirling dervishes, or the moving meditations of t'ai chi and qigong. There's even walking meditation, where the simple acts of walking and breathing become meditative. And you need not be "at peace" to meditate. Think of it this way: a still pond reflects the moon differently than a turbulent pond, but both reflect the peaceful night sky.

Meditation is about getting into more direct communication with your soul, your spirit, the universe—getting into the essence of *you* and escaping the ordinary.

Ayurvedic practitioners commonly prescribe meditation as an aspect of the healing process. There are many different kinds of meditation, and one may work better for you than another. Consulting with an Ayurvedic healer may help guide you to what type of meditation is best for you. If you don't want to, or can't, see such a healer, don't let that stop you from meditating. It's one of the most health-promoting things you can do—and it's free.

For more on meditation and yoga—an essential aspect of Ayurvedic wellness—refer to Chapter 7.

Cleansing and Detoxification—*Panchakarma*

Panchakarma is an intense form of cleansing that employs a special diet, enemas, herbal purgatives, even drinking and regurgitating salt water. (Ayurvedic cleansing is not for sissies.) There is dry brushing of the skin and sweating through exercise and in steam baths. Massages, too, using plenty of herb-infused oil, are an important element of panchakarma.

To avoid a need for more extreme measures, Ayurvedic practitioners and their patients are encouraged to pay daily attention to moving toxins out through the colon, lungs, skin, and urinary tract. There are several practices which help to achieve this.

- A pint of hot water with lemon and a pinch of salt in the morning helps keep the bowels moving. And squatting and pressing one knee at a time toward the floor with the hands helps to move the hot lemon and salt mixture through the intestines. The herb mixture *Trifala* is often used when this doesn't work.

- Frequent exercise with plenty of sweating is recommended to move toxins out through the skin. Hot yoga, known as Bikram yoga, is performed in a steaming hot room to promote this form of cleansing. Deep breathing helps expel toxins.

The following are also recommended for day-to-day cleansing:

Lymphatic System
A system of thin vessels that carry lymphatic fluid and immune cells around in the body; includes lymph nodes, which make immune cells.

• A gum massage and special Ayurvedic blotting brush to maintain gum health;

• A low-fat, high-fiber diet to keep the colon clean;

• Nasal washes with a *neti pot* to prevent nasal and sinus congestion and ear infections;

• Supporting the lymphatic system through massages or by bouncing on a mini-trampoline.

Summing Up

Ayurveda incorporates an enormous body of knowledge, much of which has existed for over 5,000 years. It's hard to imagine improving on a medical art that has been refined and applied for so long. Many of the Ayurvedic herbs are entering the mainstream and can be found on the shelves of health food stores, but beware: this healing system is just that—a *system*—and no one herb is going to have the effect that embracing the entire Ayurvedic system will have on your overall health.

For Ayurvedic products, turn to the resources section.

Availability of Ayurvedic Practitioners

Some allopathic and naturopathic physicians incorporate Ayurvedic practices successfully with other therapies, but Ayurvedic practitioners are not licensed in the United States. In India, practitioners train for five years or more to learn this healing art. You can identify an India-trained Ayurvedic doctor by the title BAMS, the Ayurvedic equivalent of M.D.

CHAPTER 9

ACUPUNCTURE AND TRADITIONAL CHINESE MEDICINE

The texts upon which traditional Chinese medicine (TCM) is based, including the *Yellow Emperor's Classic of Internal Medicine*, were authored about 5,000 years ago. They contain detailed information about the circulatory system, including that "the heart fills the pulse with blood . . . and the force of the pulse flows into the arteries and the force of the arteries ascends into the lungs." It took thousands of years, until the seventeenth century A.D., for this ancient knowledge to be discovered in Europe.

The ancient Chinese medical texts observe that the kidneys control the body's fluid levels, bone growth, and reproduction—duties that don't, at first glance, appear to be linked. It's common knowledge that the kidneys control fluid levels, but what many don't know is that these organs transform vitamin D into the form needed for proper bone growth. Modern embryology has shown that the kidneys develop from the very same fetal cells as the organs of reproduction (the ovaries and testicles). How did they know this? Impossible to say today.

With this kind of insight—developed without the techniques that have enabled contemporary medical researchers to understand the innermost workings of the human body—it is hard to dismiss TCM as less scientific than allopathic medicine. On the contrary, research tools today are providing an ever-growing body of evidence showing that TCM is effective medicine—and why.

A Whirlwind Tour of Traditional Chinese Medicine

TCM resembles other schools of natural medical thought in its belief that the body strives for balance, and that—given the right tools to gently nudge it in the right direction—it will reestablish that balance using its own resources; that every part of the body and mind is intimately connected; and that the human body and mind are, in turn, intimately connected with nature. There is no division between mental and physical health in TCM. Anxiety, depression, and neurosis are all believed to be founded in organ-system imbalances.

To maintain the body in its ideal balanced state, TCM encourages moderation and balance in diet and lifestyle. Sitting all day in an office or a car must be balanced with physical activity in the fresh air. Eating sweets must be balanced with eating bitter (this latter, however, is not easy to find in the SAD, the standard American diet). Passion must be balanced with peacefulness.

According to TCM theory, anything that is alive has a life force, or *qi* (pronounced *chee*), running through it. In the human body, qi flows along *meridians*, pathways or channels that run up and down the surface of the body, linking organs and other parts of the body with a constant stream of energy.

Scientists seeking to discover what physiological structures might correspond with the meridians have found none so far. They do not exactly correspond with the circulatory system, or the pathways of the nervous or lymph systems. What is known is that stimulating them, and the acupuncture points along them, *works*.

Yin and Yang

Qi is composed of *yin* and *yang*, two interconnected, cooperative parts. When equal, these opposing forces push against one another to maintain a dynamic state of balance. When one of them predominates, however, the qi becomes imbalanced, insufficient, or entirely interrupted. The function of the TCM remedies is to re-balance the yin and yang and get the qi properly moving through the body once again.

An imbalance of yin and yang is believed to create an opening for the invasion of pathogens such as bacteria, fungi, and viruses. Only by re-establishing proper balance can the body permanently get rid of these infectious bugs.

Yin and Yang

Yin is female, passive, cold, dark, moist, sweet, water, night. It moves toward center, conserves energy, rests to its utmost, then moves.

Yang is male, active, hot, bright, salty, dry. It moves away from center, transforms energy, moves to its utmost, then rests.

To do this, TCM doctors use remedies that include acupuncture, acupressure, cupping, moxibustion, reflexology, and herbs. The first five therapies here are used to stimulate or sedate the points where the meridians come to the skin's surface. Herbs are used for their cooling or heating qualities—most illnesses are categorized as either cold or hot in TCM, and counteracting the chill or heat of those disease states is believed to help the individual return to a balanced, healthy state. For example, the cooling herbs rhubarb and senna are both used to treat constipation, a condition of excessive heat; the hot herbs cayenne and ginger are used to treat conditions characterized in TCM by cold, such as indigestion, osteoarthritis, and poor circulation.

TCM encourages a balanced diet and lifestyle, exercise, not too much passion or activity, and time to de-stress. The practice of qigong, a form of therapeutic exercise and breathwork, is a standard self-care recommendation, and is highly beneficial for those who wish to improve their body awareness, their energy, and their health overall. (For more on qigong, refer to Chapter 7.)

Diagnosis in TCM

The TCM doctor spends years learning to make

exact and specific diagnoses of imbalances in various organs and learning to create equally specific treatment plans.

Traditionally, and as in Ayurvedic medicine, the measurement of six pulses at each wrist—three superficial and three deep—has been used to diagnose qi imbalances in TCM. (Recent research shows that these pulses do indeed have different patterns on an oscilloscope.) Unfortunately, this art is not often practiced in Chinese medicine today, as it takes too many years of study and practice to master. Now, TCM doctors usually diagnose with a *pulse generalization* instead, gauging it as reflective of either deficient or excessive qi. A tongue exam, an evaluation of the patient's smell and posture, and detailed interviews are used to gather further information.

Acupuncture

TCMs signature therapy is acupuncture. Thin needles are placed at specific points along the meridians to influence the flow of qi. The needles are used once and then disposed of, in accordance with biohazard guidelines. Various angles and motions of the needles, including plucking, raising, rotating, thrusting, twirling, or vibrating, are used to create various effects, depending on an enormously complex diagnostic decision-making process performed by the TCM doctor.

Everyone wants to know, does acupuncture hurt? It shouldn't. The needles are extremely thin and are pressed quickly into the skin. To intensify their beneficial effects, some TCM practitioners pass a current with very low power into the needles. This practice, known as *electroacupuncture*, is widely used in China for pain relief and surgical anesthesia. *Auricular* acupuncture focuses on needling the ear, which is rich in nerve endings and blood flow and is believed to have energy connections to every organ.

According to a recent consensus statement from

the National Institutes of Health, the overall body of research indicates that acupuncture may be a safe, effective treatment for:

- Addiction to alcohol, cigarettes, or hard drugs;

- Asthma;

- Carpal tunnel syndrome;

- Fibromyalgia;

- Headaches, including migraines;

- Menstrual cramps;

- Osteoarthritis;

- Post-operative, chemotherapy-induced, and pregnancy-induced nausea and vomiting;

- Post-operative dental pain;

- Stroke rehabilitation;

- Tennis elbow.

As with any natural therapy, acupuncture works best when used as part of a comprehensive program to improve overall health and encourage the body's natural tendency toward balance. And also, as with any natural therapy, acupuncture doesn't work for everyone everytime.

A good deal of research has gone into trying to figure out how acupuncture delivers its good results. Some theorize it works by altering levels of hormones, immune cells, or prostaglandins (hormone-like biochemicals). Other research suggests that acupuncture increases *endorphin* levels, the feel-good, pain-killing chemicals made in the body. Still other studies have detected alterations in neurotransmitter levels during needling, or an alteration of blood-vessel activity where needles are inserted.

Recent research has found that the acupuncture points have high electrical conductivity compared to the tissues that surround them, and they have a higher metabolic rate and temperature. People who visit a TCM doctor complaining of *myofascial pain syndrome*, a mysterious pain syndrome that is expressed in extremely tender trigger points along the body, learn that those points correspond closely with acupuncture points.

There is something special and different about the acupuncture points, and science is on the cusp of figuring out what that something is.

Acupressure

Acupressure is acupuncture without needles, performed with the fingers or using an instrument with a hard, ball-shaped head. Reflexology is acupressure performed on the ankles and feet, which are believed to contain nerve endings that link up to every part of the body.

Cupping

Cupping involves applying small glass, metal, or wooden jars to the skin, using a vacuum that is usually created by lighting a small wad of alcohol-soaked gauze inside the jar just before applying it to the skin. This vacuum draws blood to the area, which in turn stimulates the healing process. TCM practitioners may use cupping to treat backaches or soft-tissue injuries, or to help clear a buildup of excess fluid caused by chronic bronchitis. The meridians and acupuncture points provide the guidelines for where to apply the cups.

Moxibustion

This therapy is used to treat conditions related to the stagnation or cooling of qi. It involves herbs burned on or close to acupuncture points to bring heat to the area. Direct moxibustion involves the application of a small cone-shaped pile of herbs placed on the point and burned long enough to introduce pleasant warmth that penetrates the skin. Indirect moxibustion involves placing the *moxa*, as the herbs are called, on the end of an acupuncture needle that has already been introduced into the appropriate point, and burning them to deliver heat through the metal into the skin; indirect moxibustion may also use a stick of burning moxa that the TCM practitioner holds near the point being stimulated.

Moxibustion has been successfully used to turn breech babies around in the womb. Several studies support this practice as a method for avoiding Caesarian section, the usual intervention in breech births.

Moxa is used to treat arthritis, asthma, and bronchitis—all believed to be cool illnesses that are ameliorated by bringing warmth to specific acupuncture points.

For information on how to find a qualified TCM practitioner, turn to the resources section.

CHAPTER 10

NATUROPATHIC MEDICINE

Naturopathic medicine is a union and integration of natural healing modalities from around the world. It embraces ancient wisdom, traditional philosophies, and most of the natural healing practices that have shown benefit in healing or allaying suffering of humans and animals. These practices apply the forces of nature through foods, herbs, spices, hot and cold water (hydrotherapy), sunlight, and aspects of physical, biochemical, psychological, and spiritual medicine.

A doctor of naturopathic medicine will have graduated from a four-year postgraduate-level residential medical school, with extensive training in conventional medical practices, including minor surgery, pharmacy, injections, childbirthing, acupuncture, nutritional therapeutics, botanical medicine, homeopathy, physical therapy, and psychological counseling. A naturopathic doctor (N.D.) is a general family practitioner who may have areas of special interest or focus.

The Naturopathic Medical Philosophy

It is not whether a naturopathic doctor uses an herb or a homeopathic remedy or practices hydrotherapy that defines this type of health care, but rather the underlying philosophy that defines how and why a therapy is chosen and applied. Because the healing process is improved in a willing partnership, prescriptions of any kind are discussed with the patient and are written only if the patient agrees it's the best course,

A naturopathic doctor believes and follows five basic principles of healing:

1. *The Healing Power of Nature.* Nature heals powerfully through intrinsic systems in the body, mind, spirit, and soul to maintain, correct, and restore health. Naturopathic doctors work to encourage and support these inherent healing systems by using an appropriate combination of conventional and traditional medicines, methods, and techniques that are in harmony with natural healing processes.

2. *First, Do No Harm.* Naturopaths prefer non-invasive treatments that minimize the risks of harmful side effects. They are trained to distinguish who can be safely treated and who may need to be referred to another healthcare provider.

3. *Find the Cause.* Every illness has an underlying cause or causes, often involving lifestyle, diet, habits, and thoughts. A naturopathic doctor is trained to seek and address the underlying cause of a disease, not just suppress symptoms.

4. *Treat the Whole Person.* Naturopathic medicine acknowledges that health and disease come from a complex interaction of physical, emotional, dietary, genetic, environmental, and lifestyle factors.

5. *Preventive Medicine.* The naturopathic approach to health care can create health for a long and productive life and prevent minor illnesses from becoming more serious—or from becoming chronic and degenerative. Naturopathic doctors live the true meaning of the word *doctor*—"teacher"—and explain and teach healthy living and lifestyle issues to keep people vibrant and out of harm's way.

During an appointment with an N.D., expect a thorough interview about your physical and emotional health, what's going on in your life, and the environments in which you live and work. The N.D. will then map out a treatment plan with you that may integrate much of what you've read here.

If you choose to visit a naturopath as a primary healthcare practitioner, seek out an N.D. who has a degree from one of the following schools: Bastyr University just north of Seattle, Washington, the Canadian College of Naturopathic Medicine in Canada, the National College of Naturopathic Medicine in Oregon, Southwest College of Naturopathic Physicians in Tempe, Arizona, or the University of Bridgeport College of Natural Medicine in Connecticut.

Be Aware: Not All Naturopaths Are Naturopathic Doctors

An N.D. may not, in true fact, be an N.D. Confusing,

The Story of Big Ed

When Dr. Laux was a fresh-faced young N.D. and had just set up his first practice, his dad—Big Ed—fell while mowing the lawn and broke his ankle. While he was in the hospital, tests revealed a serious dangerous arrhythmia (irregular heartbeat). Soon, Big Ed was on several medications. His problems escalated, and Dr. Laux felt compelled to close his practice in Oregon to fly home and help with his father's care.

Dr. Laux was stunned when he saw his dad— bloated, gray, overweight, sleep-deprived, and bleeding under his skin from anti-clotting drugs. He immediately said, "It's the drugs that are the problem," which the cardiologist—a legend, and one of Dr. Laux's best friends although twenty-five years his senior—vigorously denied. Even though he had been practicing only a short while, Dr. Laux was convinced he had to intervene in his dad's treatment.

The cardiologist and the other allopathic doctors all believed that Big Ed had a liver tumor, which would explain the dreadful symptoms he was experiencing. Dr. Laux felt sure his dad was having nothing more complicated than a drug reaction. When he told this to the cardiologist yes, but worth making the distinction when your health is at stake. There is a difference in education between a true naturopathic physician and some others who may call themselves the same. In states where N.D.s can be licensed, there is also a big contrast between the services each can provide.

While a traditional N.D., or naturopath (not a doctor), has healing knowledge, it is frequently limited in depth and scope. The traditional naturopath usually lacks clinical training with patients, because his or her education comes from online or correspondence-school curriculums that can be completed in months. A real N.D.'s education usually entails eight years of study, including pre-med, postgradu-

---

and said he wanted to take Big Ed off all his medications, the doctor warned, "You're going to kill him," to which Dr. Laux unstintingly replied, "Better me than you." Within a few days, Big Ed was lying on the floor having acupressure treatments, with tea bags and cucumbers on his eyes.

Contrary to the cardiologist's warning, Big Ed wasn't dead within five days, he was very much alive and able to travel to Oregon with his son. And a few days after the drugs were stopped, the cardiologist called Dr. Laux to say he agreed that the problem had indeed been a negative reaction to the drugs.

In Oregon, Dr. Laux brought his dad to the hot springs twice a week and took him to the clinic for acupuncture and manipulative therapies, as well as to the gym for exercise. Visits to a tanning salon helped increase Big Ed's vitamin-D levels to aid in mending an ankle fracture he'd sustained from the fall. Big Ed lost thirty-five pounds and looked like a million bucks. The initial problem— the arrhythmia—had not been corrected, but when a new type of pacemaker came along to fix it, Big Ed was living a healthy, normal life and was ready to undergo the necessary surgery, after which he lived a full, active life for many years.

ate medical school, and clinical training—all similar to the training and education of medical doctors.

This difference provides greater scope of practice, clinical acumen, and involvement in the medical community. A naturopathic doctor/physician is a primary-care provider, and has the training and skills to diagnosis and treat most acute and chronic illness. They are trained in pharmacy prescriptions and drug protocols, natural medicine use (alone or with other medications), and laboratory tests.

A naturopathic doctor, when appropriate, makes referrals and works closely with conventional doctors to give people access to therapies and procedures outside the scope of a general family practitioner.

You can't hold a gun to a plant's flower and tell it to grow. You can, however, give it good soil and water and plenty of nutrients and protect it against deer, pest infestations, rabbits, and tromping feet. This, in essence, is the naturopathic approach. Use what works and do no harm!

For guidelines on finding a naturopathic doctor in your area, turn to the resources section.

States/Territories in Which N.D.s Are Licensed

Alaska, Arizona, California, Connecticut, Hawaii, Kansas, Maine, Montana, New Hampshire, Oregon, Puerto Rico, Utah, Vermont, Virgin Islands., Washington, Washington, D.C.

CONCLUSION

If you haven't done so already, check in with yourself now. Are you generally healthy? Do you think you are doing all you can to stay that way? If so, good for you. You might only need healthcare attention once in a great while. Using natural medical methods will help move you back toward balanced health before you fall too far from center.

Are there any illnesses you worry about developing because of family history or risky behaviors? Have you recovered from an illness you'd rather not revisit? Natural medicine excels for prevention. Learn all you can about this illness and talk with practitioners of natural therapies so you can set up a plan to protect yourself from once again losing your health.

Are you ill right now? Sometimes, being sick is all the motivation needed to get self-care and healthcare back on track—or get it on track in the first place. Your body is telling you it's time to make some changes. The guidance of natural healers will support you in doing so, and will help complement the labors of your allopathic medical team, should you need one. Increasing numbers of allopathic doctors are accepting their patients' commitments to helping themselves heal through natural means. If your doctor scoffs at your commitment to doing this, it's time to find another doctor.

Recognizing and embracing the amazing healing power of nature, you will grow to appreciate the depth of your relationship to the natural world. You, and all of us, are the stewards of that world, and only through responsible stewardship will it be possible to preserve the healing plants, foods, and other substances that are its gifts. Depending on nature to help you heal will help you, in turn, be more grateful and careful of those gifts.

SELECTED
REFERENCES

Aggarwal, BB, Kumar, A, Bharti, AC. "Anticancer potential of curcumin in preclinical and clinical studies." *Anticancer Research*, 2003; January-February 23(1A):363–398.

Ankri, S, Mirelman, D. "Antimicrobial properties of allicin from garlic." *Microbes and Infection*, 1999; February; 1(2):125–129.

Biser, JA. "Really wild remedies—medicinal plant use by animals." *Smithsonian National Zoological Park*, 1998: February.

Bland, Jeffrey, et al. *Clinical Nutrition: A Functional Approach*. The Institute for Functional Medicine, Gig Harbor, WA:1999.

Condor, Bob. "Living well: blueberries trigger neurons that keep the brain sharp." *Seattle Post-Intelligencer*, 2004; September 6.

"Curcuma longa (turmeric). Monograph." *Alternative Medicine Review*, 2001; September; 6 Suppl:S62–66.

Fleischauer, AT, Arab, L. "Garlic and Cancer: A Critical Review of the Epidemiologic Literature." *Journal of Nutrition*, 2001; 131:1032–1040S.

Fletcher, RK, Fairfield, Kathleen. "Vitamins for Chronic Disease Prevention in Adults: Clinical Applications." *Journal of the American Medical Association (JAMA)*, 2002; June 19; 287(23):3127–3129.

Goel, V, et al. "Efficacy of a standardized echinacea preparation (Echinilin) for the treatment of the common cold: a randomized, double-blind, placebo-controlled trial." *International Journal of Clinical Pharmacology and Therapeutics*, 2004; February; 29(1):75–83.

Gross, AP, et al. "A Cochrane review of manipulation and mobilization for mechanical neck disorders." *Spine*, 2004 ; July15; 29(14):1541–1548.

Homola, Samuel. "What a rational chiropractor can do for you." Chirobase, August 22, 2003, www.chirobase.org.

Kiefer, David, Pantuso, Traci. "Panax ginseng." *American Family Physician,* 2003; October 15, www.aafp.org/afp/20031015/1539.html.

Muller, PS, Plevak, DJ, Rummans,TA. "Religious involvement, spirituality, and medicine: implications for clinical practice." *Mayo Clinic Proceedings,* 2001 December; 76(12):1225–1235.

National Institutes of Health Consensus Development Statement, "Acupuncture." 1997; November 3–5.

Rabe, A, Weiser, M, Klein, P. "Effectiveness and tolerability of a homoeopathic remedy compared with conventional therapy for mild viral infections." *International Journal of Clinical Practice,* 2004; Sep; 58(9):827–832.

"Siberian ginseng." Herb Library at HealthCentral.com. *The People's Pharmacy Guide to Home and Herbal Remedies* by Joe and Teresa Graedon (St. Martin's Press, 1999.)

Sierpina, VS, Wollschlaeger, B, Blumenthal, M. "Ginkgo biloba."*American Family Physician,* 2003; September 1; 68(5):923–926.

Vita, JA. "Polyphenols and cardiovascular disease: effects on endothelial and platelet function." *American Journal of Clinical Nutrition,* 2005; January; 81(1 Suppl): 2925–2975.

Wasser, SP. "Review of medical mushrooms advances: good news for old allies." *HerbalGram,* 2002; 56:28–33.

Yao, LH, et al. "Flavonoids in food and their health benefits." *Plant Foods and Human Nutrition,* 2004; Summer; 59(3):113–122.

Zapatero, JM. "Selections from current literature: effects of hawthorn on the cardiovascular system." *Family Practice,* 1999; 16(5):534–538.

OTHER BOOKS
AND RESOURCES

Acupuncture and Traditional Chinese Medicine

Websites

American Association of Oriental Medicine:
1-888-500-7999 or www.aaom.org
For information on acupuncture and TCM. Members are recognized as highly qualified TCM practitioners.

National Certification Commission for Acupuncture and Oriental Medicine (NCCAOM):
www.nccaom.org/find.htm
Lists TCM practitioners. Seek out one who holds a Diploma of Oriental Medicine (Dipl. O.M.) or a Diploma of Acupuncture (Dipl. Ac.).

American Academy of Medical Acupuncturists (AAMA):
www.medicalacupuncture.org/aama_marf/aama.html
If you feel more comfortable with an acupuncturist who is trained in Western medicine, go here, but be aware that these doctors may lack the in-depth skills of the acupuncturists who have trained for years in China, where acupuncture originated.

Ayurvedic Medicine

Website

Banyan Botanicals: www.banyanbotanicals.com
To find Ayurvedic herbs and neti pots. Also check with your local health food store.

Healing Diets and Superfoods

Books

Living Cuisine: The Art and Spirit of Raw Foods by J. Underkoffer (Avery Health Guides, 2003).

Rainbow Green Live Food Cuisine by Gabriel Cousens, M.D. (North Atlantic Books, 2003).

The Macrobiotic Path to Total Health: A Complete Guide to Preventing and Relieving More than 200 Chronic Conditions by Michio Kushi and Alex Jack (Ballantine Books, 2003).

The New Whole Foods Encyclopedia: A Comprehensive Resource for Healthy Eating by Rebecca Wood (Penguin Books, 1999).

Whole Foods Companion: A Guide for Adventurous Cooks, Curious Shoppers, and Lovers of Natural Foods by Dianne Onstad (Chelsea Green Publishing Company, 2005).

Websites

Gourmet Mushrooms and Mushroom Products: www.gmushrooms.com
This is an online mail-order source for dried medicinal mushrooms.

The Kushi Institute: www.kushiinstitute.org/newsletter/mbr.pdf
Website has detailed macrobiotic guidelines.

Herbal Medicine

Book
The Green Pharmacy Herbal Handbook by James A. Duke (Rodale Inc., 2000).

Websites

HealthCentral.com: www.healthcentral.com/peoplespharmacy/peoplespharmacy.cfm
Joe and Theresa Graedon, a pharmacologist and a medical anthropologist, are well-known for their People's Pharmacy books. Their site is an excellent resource for up-to-date herb and supplement news.

Herb Research Foundation: www.herbs.org
A great resource for unbiased, science-based information.

University of Maryland Medical Center: www.umm.edu/altmed/ConsLookups/Herbs.html
This site has an extensive database of medicinal herbs and good, research-based information.

Homeopathy

Book

Radical Healing: Integrating the World's Great Therapeutic Traditions to Create A New Transformative Medicine by Rudolph Ballentine, M.D. (Three Rivers Press, 1999).

An excellent reference on homeopathic self-care by the director of the Center for Holistic Medicine in New York City.

Website

Council for Homeopathic Certification: www.homeopathicdirectory.com
Good place to find a licensed homeopathic practitioner in your area. Try to find an M.D., D.O., registered nurse, N.D., or D.C. who holds one of these certifications.

Manipulative Therapies— Chiropractic and Osteopathic

Websites

Chirobase: www.chirobase.org
This organization has a referral list of chiropractors who agree with its very conservative guidelines. Your health insurer may offer coverage for chiropractic. Try to get a referral from your general practitioner or from trusted friends or relatives.

American Osteopathic Association: 1-800-621-1773 or www.osteopathic.org
Can help you find an osteopath near you.

Massage Therapy and Bodywork

Website

The American Massage Therapy Association: 1-888-843-2682 or www.amtamassage.org
AMTA has a nationwide list of practitioners who are certified at the national level.

Mind/Body Work

Books

Anatomy of an Illness by Norman Cousins (W.W. Norton, 1979).

Full Catastrophe Living by Jon Kabat-Zinn, M.D. (Dell Publishing, 1990).

A good introduction to meditation for beginners.

Wellness Workbook: How to Achieve Enduring Health and Vitality, 3rd Edition by John W. Travis, M.D. and Regina Sara Ryan (Celestial Arts, Berkeley/Toronto, 2004).

A simple, comprehensive approach to mind/body/feeling integration as a path to wellness.

Websites

The Coach Connection:
www.findyourcoach.com/discover-coaching-lvl1.htm

Transcendental Meditation, the Maharishi Vedic Education Development Corporation:
1-888-532-7686 or www.tm.org

World Prayers: www.worldprayers.org
A multicultural prayer archive to find ideas for prayer.

Naturopathic Medicine

Website

American Association of Naturopathic Practitioners:
1-866-538-2267 or www.naturopathic.org
Lists naturopathic physicians and provides information.

Nutritional Supplements

Books

Comparative Guide to Nutritional Supplements by Lyle McWilliam (Northern Dimensions Publishing, 2003).

Feed Your Genes Right: Eat to Turn Off Disease-Causing Genes and Slow Down Aging by Jack Challem. (John Wiley and Sons, 2005).

Prescription for Nutritional Healing: The A to Z Guide to Supplements by James Balch and Phyllis Balch (Avery Books, 2002).

Websites

ConsumerLab.com:
www.consumerlab.com/index.asp
An independent testing agency that evaluates nutritional supplements.

Dietary Supplement Information Bureau:
www.supplementinfo.org
A supplement industry group.

Dr. Marcus Laux: www.drmarcuslaux.com

Life Extension Foundation: www.lef.org

Linus Pauling Institute: www.lpi.oregonstate.edu

National Institutes for Health: www.nccam.nih.gov
This is the NIH alternative medicine site.

GreatLife Magazine
Consumer magazine with articles on vitamins, minerals, herbs, and foods.
Available for free at many health and natural food stores.

Let's Live Magazine
Consumer magazine with emphasis on the health benefits of vitamins, minerals, and herbs.
Customer service:
1-800-676-4333
P.O. Box 74908
Los Angeles, CA 90004
Subscriptions: 12 issues per year, $19.95 in the U.S.; $31.95 outside the U.S.

Physical Magazine
Magazine oriented to body builders and other serious athletes.
Customer service:
1-800-676-4333
P.O. Box 74908
Los Angeles, CA 90004
Subscriptions: 12 issues per year, $19.95 in the U.S.; $31.95 outside the U.S.

The Nutrition Reporter™ newsletter
Monthly newsletter that summarizes recent medical research on vitamins, minerals, and herbs.
Customer service:
P.O. Box 30246
Tucson, AZ 85751-0246
e-mail: jack@thenutritionreporter.com
www.nutritionreporter.com
Subscriptions: $26 per year (12 issues) in the U.S.; $32 U.S. or $48 CNC for Canada; $38 for other countries

INDEX